The

E

| | | DATE DUE | | |
|---|---|---|---|
| | | | |
| | | | |
| | | | |
| | | | |
| | | | |
| | | | |
| | | | |
| | | | |
| | | | |
| | | | |
| | | | |
| | | | |

# The
# Eldercare
## Sourcebook

JOAN C. BREITUNG, R.N., M.A., M.S.N.

***Contemporary Books***

Chicago   New York   San Francisco   Lisbon   London   Madrid   Mexico City
Milan   New Delhi   San Juan   Seoul   Singapore   Sydney   Toronto

**Library of Congress Cataloging-in-Publication Data**

Breitung, Joan Carson.
      The eldercare sourcebook / Joan Carson Breitung.
         p.    cm.
      Includes bibliographical references.
      ISBN 0-658-01657-1
      1. Aged.    2. Aged—Care.    I. Title.

HQ1061 .B716    2002
305.26—dc21                  2001047587

*Contemporary Books*

A Division of The *McGraw·Hill* Companies

1 2 3 4 5 6 7 8 9 0   AGM/AGM   1 0 9 8 7 6 5 4 3 2

ISBN 0-658-01657-1

This book was set in Sabon
Printed and bound by Quebecor Martinsburg

McGraw-Hill books are available at special quantity discounts to use as premiums and sales promotions, or for use in corporate training programs. For more information, please write to the Director of Special Sales, Professional Publishing, McGraw-Hill, Two Penn Plaza, New York, NY 10121-2298. Or contact your local bookstore.

This book is printed on acid-free paper.

*To Ben*
*L'chayim!*

# Contents

# Introduction

THE GLOBAL POPULATION is at an all-time high and is rapidly increasing. This fact alone raises concern because of the serious social, economic, and political problems that are the consequences of overpopulation. However, the most ominous aspect of current population trends is the percentage represented by the elderly—adults over sixty-five—whose numbers are increasing at a much higher rate than any other age group.

In 1950 the population of the world's elderly was 200 million. This figure will rise to 1.2 billion by 2025, a sixfold increase in only seventy-five years. The most significant increase in elder longevity is found, unsurprisingly, in developed countries. By the year 2025, one out of four people in the developed world will be sixty years of age or older. This very large population of elderly persons will have the financial resources and political influence to demand quality care when the need arises.

The most pressing problem to result from this exponentially rapid growth in our elderly population will be the need for a substantial increase in the numbers of health care professionals and the services they provide. At present, there is a serious shortage of clinicians specifically trained in geriatrics. In 1992 there were only 4,000 geriatricians to provide care for 30 million elderly people—just 1.32 geriatricians for every 10,000 Americans aged sixty-five or older. The busy primary-care physician is the first line of defense. Other resources also are strained. The nursing profession has experienced its fifth consecutive year of declining student enrollment, and there is a national shortage of pharmacists. The data explicit in the U.S. Census tell the story. The population numbers and the warning they are sounding are clear.

With a shortage of professionals, who will be there to provide care for the elderly? About 5 percent of the elderly are in nursing homes, where they are cared for by a dwindling number of trained caregivers. The other 95 percent are living in the community. Some frail elderly are the responsibility of their adult children, often members of the pressured "sandwich generation," those who, while employed, struggle to meet the needs of their own families and of their impaired parents. Others are cared for by spouses, who typically are managing their own infirmities. Many other older adults, generally widows, live alone.

If our present professional elder care services are already critically and often dangerously strained, what will the situation be when the 76 million baby boomers in the United States reach old age and demand quality care for their mounting medical needs? *The Elder Care Sourcebook*, a valuable resource for caregivers, the health professionals who work with them, and the elderly themselves can provide a starting point for everyone seeking more information. It gives individuals and their families facing the problems associated with aging a more positive and constructive experience in solving such problems.

The book begins with background information on population trends and future directions in aging. Next, Chapter 2 summarizes the state of current thinking about the aging process, in terms of biological change and changes in a person's psychological and interpersonal experiences. Chapter 3 outlines the nutritional needs of the elderly person, as well as signs of malnutrition. Because the elderly tend to be the heaviest users of over-the-counter and prescription medications, they are at greater risk for problems associated with drug use. Chapter 4 therefore explores the most common and serious pharmacological problems, including noncompliance with medication plans and side effects of drug use. Chapter 5 addresses the myths and realities of sexuality in the aging person, and it provides some guidelines for healthy sexual expression in this population.

Although older adults are living longer and healthier lives, this population is at greater risk for illness, institutionalization, and death. Chapter 6 discusses common problems with mental health, especially depression and dementia. The concerns of elder abuse and ageism are the topic of Chapter 7, which identifies symptoms and solutions to these problems. Chapter 8 covers types of long-term care facilities and issues that the elderly and their caregivers should address in order to make a successful transition to long-term care. Chapter 9 discusses resources for coping with dying and bereavement, from successful coping at the personal level to the use of hospice services.

The last chapter addresses our society's conflicting assumptions about aging and the quality of life. Some think that because people are living longer, the general health of the elderly must be good. Others hold the view that all old people are frail and sick. The truth lies somewhere in between, and Chapter 10 interprets the older adults' unique health needs. Throughout all the chapters, *The Elder Care Sourcebook* explains the physical and psychological aspects of aging and suggests ways of optimizing the strengths of older adults. Following the chapters, five appendixes present lists of suggested books and videos, as well as a broad range of organizations and support services.

Old age can be rewarding. If the elderly, their caregivers, and their families are prepared and informed, they can work cooperatively with health care professionals to make beneficial choices and constructive decisions. In doing so, they make the lives of frail older adults safer and more comfortable.

# 1

# The Aging Population

PEOPLE TYPICALLY THINK of the United States as a young nation. In 1900 the country's elderly population, persons over the age of sixty-five, was only 4.1 percent of the general population. During the next fifty years, however, the elderly population doubled to about 8 percent. In 1994, only forty-four years later, the percentage of people over age sixty-five was 12 percent. Amazingly, the percentage of the elderly in America has tripled in one century.

The subset within the elderly population known as the "oldest old," persons aged eighty-five and over, had the largest percentage increase in longevity among the elderly population. One of the chief factors contributing to this longer life expectancy was the significant decline in mortality, especially from heart disease. Death rates from heart disease among persons sixty-five to eighty-four have fallen by about half since 1970, and among those aged eighty-five and over, death rates from heart disease have dropped 21 percent.

Another reason for the population increase in the elderly age group is the very high rate of immigration from Europe that occurred during the first decade of the twentieth century, accompanied by continued high levels of births. Between 1900 and 1910, almost 30 percent of the population growth in the United States resulted from immigration. This had a significant effect on the population, since developed countries have relatively low rates of fertility and mortality.

*Population growth is concentrated among baby boomers (persons born between 1946 and 1964) and the elderly. Baby boomers are about 30 percent of the population. At present, adults over age sixty-five (the elderly) are 13 percent.*

In spite of longer life expectancy and declining mortality rates for the population as a whole, the number of elderly deaths continued to rise during the 1990s. The major reason for that increase has been the age structure of the population. High growth in the population of the oldest old has produced a larger population in age categories with the greatest likelihood of dying. As long as the oldest-old group keeps growing, the number of deaths will continue to increase each year unless the age-specific death rates in this population sharply decline.

## Differences for Men and Women

In 1998 there were 20.2 million older women and 14.2 million older men, or 143 women for every 100 men. The ratio of women to men increases with age. Among those aged sixty-five to sixty-nine, the ratio is 118 to 100, and among those eighty-five and over, there are 241 women for every 100 men. These figures provide impressive evidence of women's greater longevity.

Not only do women as a group live longer than men, they are more likely to survive the illnesses that are major causes of death. The reasons are unclear, and science still has not determined a fundamental, biologic cause for the difference in life expectancy between the genders.

Although men are more vulnerable than women to most causes of death, particularly cardiovascular disease, cardiovascular disease has made significant inroads into women's well-being in recent decades. Cardiovascular disease, and in particular coronary heart disease, remains the leading cause of death in both men and women sixty-five years and older. A growing proportion of women have coronary heart disease, partly because better treatment means they are less likely to die as a result (so they are more likely to live with it) and partly as a result of longer life expectancy (so they are more likely to live long enough to experience coronary heart disease).

A clear trend toward longer life expectancy for women emerged in the beginning of the twentieth century. Before then, childbirth was so hazardous that women often died, so women's and men's life expectancies were nearly equal. Along with improved health care during pregnancy and childbirth, other developments have since improved female longevity. Modern women have benefited from overall improvements in health care, work opportunities, and athletic activity.

Men have a higher death rate than do women at every age. This difference increases with advancing age. Consequently, while most elderly men are married, most elderly women are widows.

*In 1998 almost half of all women over sixty-five years of age were widows. There were four times as many widows as widowers in this age group.*

The age advantage for women is a mixed blessing, since for women there are many more years in which to experience the inevitable chronic diseases, functional limitations, and social losses. While most elderly men have a spouse for assistance when their health declines, most elderly women do not. Elderly women are much more likely than elderly men to live alone, a difference that steadily increases with age.

Elderly women also have a higher poverty rate than elderly men—16 percent versus 9 percent, or nearly twice as high. They are a special subgroup within the population of the elderly poor. Depending on their employment history, elderly women are likely either to have an inadequate pension plan or no pension plan when they reach their retirement years. In addition, many elderly women have had to exhaust their own pensions or the income and benefits they were entitled to receive from their husbands' pensions when it became necessary to provide long-term medical care for the husband.

# Cultural Differences

Although whites now dominate the elderly population, their relative numbers are projected to decline over the next sixty years as the numbers of ethnic minority elderly increase. In 1980 members of ethnic minority groups represented a little more than 10 percent of the elderly population. In 1990 this figure rose to slightly over 13 percent, and they are projected to be one-third of the elderly population by 2050. The black older-adult population increased by about 20 percent from 1980 to 1990, compared with a 57 percent increase for Hispanics and a 150 percent Asian-American increase in the same time period.

The elderly population is one of the most diverse and ethnically varied groups in the United States. Understanding, predicting, and improving level of functioning and quality of life among minority elders are firmly tied to social and cultural circumstances. These older adults have a broad array of histories, cultural beliefs and practices, languages, and health care needs. Their circumstances range from being totally self-sufficient to requiring minimal supervision and in-home services, and, finally, to depending upon twenty-four-hour skilled nursing care.

Cultural factors play an important role in health care. Culture—the combination of behavior patterns, beliefs, and institutions that are typical of a population or community—affects all aspects of illness, including the following:

- *Risk factors*—American Indians and Alaskan Natives are at high risk for diabetes. African-Americans bear a relatively great risk for hypertension.
- *Beliefs about the causes and the course of an illness*—Some cultures believe that illness is a punishment from God, and that an improved relationship with God will affect the course of the illness. A visit to a church service or attention of a minister may be the first step in attempting to solve a health problem.
- *Compliance with treatment recommendations*—Among Mexican-Americans, health is traditionally viewed as the

absence of pain. Therefore, in that context, if a person is not in pain, there is no illness.

The Older Americans Act, a federal focal point which created the Administration on Aging (an advocacy agent for the elderly), was amended in 1987. The amendments focused national attention on the needs of minority groups by mandating that services be targeted to those in greatest social and economic need, particularly minority elderly. The minority elderly referred to are generally identified as Asian/Pacific Islander, Native American, Hispanic, or African-American.

These four categories of non-European populations can help us identify cultural differences, but the categories are far from perfect. One limitation is that each group has a diverse and heterogeneous membership. For example, the category Asian/Pacific Islander includes such distinct ancestries as Korean, Japanese, Chinese, Filipino, and Samoan. Native Americans comprise several hundred tribes and reservations, including American Indians, Aleuts, and Inuits. Members of the Hispanic group may share a common language and some cultural traditions, but there are many differences among Puerto Rican, Cuban, Latin American, Mexican, and Central American populations. Elderly African-Americans also have many distinguishing characteristics related to the geographic regions in which they live, their rural and urban lifestyles, and different socioeconomic conditions. These differences require that health care professionals be aware of heterogeneity within and among cultural groups in order to avoid stereotyping.

Another drawback with these definitions of four ethnic minority categories is that the designations, while generally accepted, are sometimes arbitrary. For example, demographers view Native Hawaiians as an Asian/Pacific Islander group, but Title VI of the Older Americans Act includes them in the category of Native American/Alaskan Natives.

In spite of these drawbacks, the categories help us to identify areas of need. Elderly adults of color have been found to be slightly more likely than other elderly persons to experience psychosocial distress. This is especially true for those who have lived in poverty, are under-educated, live in substandard housing, and lack opportunity. Under these circumstances, the occasions to cultivate social and psychological resources are remote.

At the same time, some experts have questioned the accuracy of reports of psychiatric illnesses among African-Americans. Some researchers have found biases in diagnosing such illness. One glaring example has been a more frequent diagnosis of schizophrenia among blacks than was shown to be valid. Reasons for the errors ranged from racism to nonblack psychiatrists' lack of rapport with and understanding of their African-American patients. As a result of these errors, restraints, both physical and chemical, were prescribed more often for elderly black patients than for elderly white patients.

Another cultural difference involves the effectiveness of nonprofessional, informal support systems in helping members of minority populations cope with mental health problems. One study, for example, concluded that family help was effective in promoting mental health for elderly blacks. However, in the same study they found that increased family interaction was associated with increased depression among elderly Mexican-Americans.

Elderly minority women share several traits with *all* elderly women. They outnumber elderly minority men. They are more likely to be widowed than elderly men of color. The longer they live, the greater the probability they will experience chronic illness, disability, and dependence. However, aged minority women bring to their later years the cumulative effects on their health of being a minority in a society in which they often faced disadvantages for this very reason. These disadvantages are reflected in the limited resources available throughout their lives to meet health care and other needs.

## Poverty Among the Elderly

In the recent past, there has been a marked increase in government and private programs to assist the indigent elderly:

- Social Security provides cost-of-living increases to recipients based on the consumer price index.
- Supplemental Social Security benefits are available to the eligible elderly and to the blind and disabled.

- The federal Medicare program provides the elderly with low-cost assistance to meet the expenses of hospital and doctor bills.
- State Medicaid programs provide other health services, such as payment for long-term care and assistance in paying for prescriptions.
- Employee pension plans now often provide residual payments to elderly women when their husbands die.
- Federal and state governments encourage planning for retirement security through favored tax plans, such as individual retirement accounts (IRAs), tax sheltered annuities (TSAs), and 401(K) plans.

These programs have been responsible for a 10.8 percent decrease in the numbers of aged poor between 1966 and 1996. In spite of these programs, however, the problem of the elderly poor remains a major concern. The improvement so far has been only modest, and the large number of elderly poor persists.

Several trends have contributed to this continued problem and concern over the elderly poor. Older adults are living longer. At the same time, the medical costs of this group are rising. The prospects of requiring long-term care are distinct threats to financial security.

Among women, the events of marriage and employment seem to distinguish younger from older women in poverty. Being married and getting a job tend to reduce the poverty rate among young women, while losing a spouse who was the major source of support, retiring from a job, or having to pay for the costs of failing health in old age increases the risk of poverty for elderly women. Furthermore, when older women become poor, they are likely to remain poor, since marriage and employment are less viable options for them as a route out of poverty.

Because women of color are more likely than white women in all age groups to be the sole head of the household and because female-headed households are more likely than households headed by males to be poor, these women are especially at risk for poverty. As minority women age and become widowed, the incidence of poverty among this group increases. Although the poverty rate among the elderly has declined, poverty is still more common for elderly women than for elderly men. In addition, within elderly ethnic minorities, poverty has increased more rapidly than it has for nonminorities.

# The Oldest Old

In the past, populations were usually divided into three major age groups: people under twenty, working-age populations (about twenty to sixty-five), and those over sixty-five. Now, however, because the population eighty-five and over has grown substantially, this group has been designated as a separate demographic entity by social scientists and the Census Bureau. People who are at least eighty-five years old represent the fourth age group—the "oldest old."

## *Impact on Society*

Never before have so many people in the United States lived so long. The proportion of the population classified as the oldest old will continue to grow. Current generations, both young and old, will be profoundly influenced by this trend. The growing population of the oldest old is redistributing educational status, increasing our society's demand for the services of caretakers, fueling political conflict between the generations, and blurring the transition from maturity to old age.

The educational divide between young and old is slowly diminishing. Today's baby boomers are the best-educated generation in our history. They are employed in an ideal economic climate, are well informed, and can be demanding when it comes to services. Where it is uncommon to see an eighty-five-year-old college graduate today, forty years from now, a college degree will be a standard characteristic of aged persons.

The potential supply of caretakers is eroding. Young people can expect to spend almost as many years caring for an elderly parent as raising their own children. The decline in potential caretakers occurred because of changes in family structure such as the increase in childless couples, single-parent families, and delayed childbearing.

Perceived generational needs are divisive. The one United Nations study revealed that the elderly are often viewed as dependent beneficiaries of economic development, rather than contributors to it. This viewpoint leads to the attitude that the elderly are not only obstacles to economic development but also societal burdens that divert needed resources away from other age groups.

The demarcation of phases that indicate the passage from adulthood to old age has become less clearly defined. Traditional characteristics of adulthood were education, marriage, and work. One of the most significant markers of approaching old age was retirement from work. However, the concept that a worker who reached the midsixties would slow down, relax, spend more time with grandchildren, and probably stop working altogether has changed. Older adults are working longer, partly because of financial concerns, but also partly because they are healthier, more vigorous as a group, and find work stimulating. The issue of second careers takes on new meaning for compulsive workers who have many years remaining.

## Who Are the Oldest Old?

The group of adults over eighty-five have distinct demographic and social differences that have implications for planning and policy issues of advanced aging. For example, people who survive to advanced old age generally have the advantages of genetics, favorable socioeconomic status, and environmental factors.

Issues dealing with advanced aging are often considered women's issues, because women dominate this age group. In the 1990 census, 1.5 million women were eighty-five years of age and older, and 675,000 men had reached the same milestone. The main reasons that women live longer than men are that men have a higher death rate from heart disease and tend to adopt certain high-risk behaviors. (However, the men who reach the eighty-five and over group have fewer chronic diseases than men who died before or at age eighty-five. Women over eighty-five who have lost spouses probably have experienced widowhood at a younger age and thus have had time to adjust to the loss of a spouse and to form relationships with other elderly women. In addition, women have been accustomed to domestic roles and family responsibility, so they have greater role continuity in late-life relationships and activities.

Besides spousal relationships, women over eighty-five have their closest associations with their children. Although grandchildren, nieces, and nephews may provide emotional support, they seldom are responsible for supervising the activities of the elderly relative. The linchpin of the support system is the adult child, traditionally adult daughters. Therefore, the death of an adult child is devastating practically as well as emotionally. About one-third of the oldest old have experienced the death of a child.

Significant differences exist between the very old who are involved with their families and those who lack family support. Because many of the oldest old have outlived spouses, siblings, and close friends, their family relationships are with younger generations. Family support, when available, ranges from financial assistance to emotional support—such as frequent telephone calls and visits—to assistance with a variety of activities of daily living such as monitoring medications, managing personal finances, shopping, and meal preparation.

## Gender Differences of the Oldest Old

Census data show some differences between the experiences of women and men among the oldest old:

- Men eighty-five and older had a higher income from all sources than did women.
- In this age group, 50 percent of the men and 10 percent of the women were married.
- Men's rate of remarriage after being widowed is seven times higher than that of women.
- Women are much more likely to be widowed than men are.
- Women are more likely than men to face a period of diminished functional capacity without spousal care.
- More women than men live alone.

Most gender-based differences fall into the categories of functional status, socioeconomic status, and social resources.

Functional differences occur because men in this age group tend to have fewer chronic diseases. Women have greater physical disabilities arising from chronic health conditions such as arthritis and osteoporosis, which deplete energy and limit mobility.

As noted earlier, women have more economic problems than men do. During the years men were working, they earned more money on average than women did. Men's benefits and retirement pensions were also more favorable. Therefore, women's average incomes are lower then men's, and retirement benefits for women also are lower.

The most notable difference in social resources occurs because women over eighty-five were typically widowed at a younger age than men in this group. By the time they reach the age of eighty-five, women have therefore had a longer time to adapt to living alone. Elderly women also tend to have more experience with domestic responsibilities and with developing self-sufficiency. Very old men usually are unprepared to manage all the household tasks, care for an impaired spouse, or deal with the stress of living alone.

## Effects of Resources

The many activities of daily living can directly affect the quality of life of the very aged individual. Managing routine chores consumes energy and leaves little in reserve to deal with the stresses and strains of everyday life. For example, if an older adult has a mobility limitation that makes it difficult to go outside the home alone, the limitation takes a psychological as well as a physical toll. The person will have difficulty maintaining social ties, and this reduces the person's quality of life.

The damaging life events that the oldest old are most likely to experience are the illness or death of a spouse and significant change in their own health. Visual and hearing impairments, for example, can severely limit a person's ability to care for basic needs, meet transportation needs, and maintain social activities. In contrast, those who have aged energetically and with enthusiasm report greater numbers of social contacts, better physical health, manageable visual and hearing impairments, and fewer threatening life events.

Common misconceptions about individuals of advanced age are that they are all alike and that their age will inevitably produce decline and a need for placement in a nursing home. The truth, however, is that there is wide variability in this population. Some people in this age group will benefit from the protective environment of a nursing home. Others can maintain a high level of functioning with forms of assistance that allow them to remain in the community and direct their own activities. People who can function at that level tend to be those with mobility—that is, they can move around indoors and out, get in and out of bed, and go up and down stairs.

These differences aside, it is certain that, as more and more of the population lives long enough to experience multiple chronic illnesses and the resulting dependency, many more relatives in their fifties and sixties will be responsible for their care. Increasing numbers of people will have to provide care for very old, frail relatives.

### Longer Life and the Compression of Morbidity

For the growing population of those living very long lives, what is the likelihood of being healthy and vigorous in advanced years, rather than disabled because of disease? The answer is unknown. One possibility, known as *compression of morbidity*, refers to the theoretical view that with healthier lifestyles, better disease prevention, and improved medications and treatment, the time span between disability and death shrinks to fewer years, even as the total life span increases.

# Availability of Health Care

As the elderly population has grown, *gerontology*, the science of describing the changes of normal aging and distinguishing them from disease effects, is becoming more sophisticated, and its value more widely recognized. In addition, *geriatrics*, the care of older adults with clinical problems, is becoming increasingly specialized. Nevertheless, there is a dearth of prepared professionals to meet the medical needs of the burgeoning aged population.

In 1993 only 8 of the nation's 126 medical schools required sep- arate courses in geriatric medicine. There were only 4,000 board- certified geriatricians to care for 30 million elderly people. The reasons for these shortages are many and varied:

- Geriatric medicine lacks the perceived stimulation and excite- ment of other specialties.
- Geriatrics is not as lucrative as other areas in medicine.

- Compared to other specialists, geriatricians less often experience the professional satisfaction of curing illness and saving lives. Rather, irreversible physical decline and death are the eventual long-term outcomes of a geriatric patient.
- Aged patients are typically covered by Medicare and other government-run programs, which often fail to pay promptly.
- There is a lack of professional role models.
- Doctors, like others in our society, are subject to negative stereotypes of aging.

Like medical schools, schools of nursing are also gradually adjusting curricula to provide appropriately prepared caregivers for the elderly. Hospitals are no longer the main locations for student nurses' clinical experience. Since geriatric patients now receive care in several sites, nurses' training can be varied. Geriatric patients now account for

- 80 percent of home visits
- 60 percent of ambulatory adult care visits (which take place at walk-in clinics)
- 85 percent of nursing home residents
- 48 percent of hospital patients

Even though the elderly are a sizable share of patients, only one in three baccalaureate nursing programs has faculty prepared to teach gerontological nursing, and only one in four schools requires a separate course in gerontology. Typically, the faculties of nursing schools defend this position by stating that gerontology is integrated into other courses, and that their curriculum is already overloaded. Gerontology thus remains a small nursing specialty. Less than 0.5 percent of all registered nurses have credentials as gerontological nurses or are prepared in the specialty at the master's or doctoral level.

# Long-Term Care

Most elderly have at least one chronic illness, and many have several medical conditions. Elderly persons accounted for 40 percent of all hospital stays in 1998 and averaged more contacts with doctors than adults under the age of sixty-five. That same year, 12 percent of the total expenditures of elderly persons were allocated to health costs—more than three times the amount spent by younger adults. Strategies and interventions to prevent disease and the resulting disabilities are necessary to control the costs of medical care incurred by those living very long lives. Even more important is the chance to improve the quality of those lives. As more people live long enough to experience multiple chronic illnesses, disability, and dependency, more relatives in their fifties and sixties will face the concern and expense of caring for this group of elders.

The need for personal assistance with everyday activities such as dressing, eating, and toileting may indicate a need for health and social services. This need typically increases with a person's age. In a 1996 study of noninstitutionalized elderly persons, 29 percent of persons aged sixty-five to seventy-five reported a need for personal assistance, compared to 75 percent of those aged eighty-five and older.

Long-term care developed as a response to the needs of impaired elderly persons by offering a variety of settings for their care. These settings range from in-home services for older adults who require some help with everyday household tasks to skilled nursing care and round-the-clock supervision for nursing home residents. The continuum of long-term care includes the following types of services:

- *Adult day care*—An adult day-care program provides health and social services for elderly adults who have physical or cognitive disabilities and need the services provided in a structured, protective setting for a few hours a day, several days each week. Some adult day-care programs offer personal care and grooming along with socializing activities designed to delay nursing home placement. The groups are small, usually no more than twenty clients at a time. Participation enables families to continue to care for an impaired family member at home, and it permits the older adult to remain in the community.
- *Home care*—As the name implies, home care takes place in the older adult's home. Homemaker/home health aides and

chore services assist with bathing, dressing, toileting, shopping, and housekeeping. Some agencies offer rehabilitative services. The advantage of home care is that it may be a practical alternative to institutionalization, allowing the elderly client to continue to live at home.

- *Respite care*—With respite care, a substitute caregiver provides family caregivers temporary relief for a few hours or a few days. Respite care may take place in a client's home or may involve moving the patient to a residential facility.
- *Supportive housing*—Although many people think of supportive housing as assisted living, the term is a collective title that may refer to foster group housing, congregate living, and retirement communities.
- *Continuing care retirement communities*—A continuing care retirement community is a housing facility that includes the entire spectrum of long-term care. Residents usually live independently, choose from a menu of services previously agreed upon, and are guaranteed life care, which includes twenty-four-hour supervision and skilled nursing care when needed.
- *Nursing homes*—Usually nursing homes are the first facilities that come to mind when a person thinks of long-term care. They are often the choice for an individual who is too frail or too cognitively impaired to be cared for at home. Nursing homes provide twenty-four-hour supervision and skilled nursing care. Some nursing homes have also developed sub-acute units, which are comprehensive inpatient settings for patients whose illnesses or injuries are stable yet require care that is more complex than conventional nursing homes can manage. When patients in sub-acute units have completed their therapies, they usually return to their own homes.
- *Foster care*—With this alternative to nursing homes, each client has his or her own room, receives all meals, is taken to medical appointments, and is supervised when taking medications. The provider is also a source of emotional support. Every state has a program for dependent adults, but state requirements and reimbursements vary widely. Nationally,

about 100,000 adults are in foster care. Approximately half are elderly, and the other half are younger adults with disabilities.

- *Hospice care*—Hospice care provides care and comfort for terminally ill persons, many of whom are older adults. Some of the benefits include nursing care (which may take place in a nursing home, hospital, or the patient's own home), home health aide services, physician's services, and bereavement counseling. Hospice care does not provide invasive procedures or heroic treatments. Rather, it offers elderly patients comfort care and a means of dying with dignity.

- *Access services*—Within the field of long-term care, access services help older adults identify and obtain other services such as transportation, information, and referral. Transportation is a major problem for many elderly who live in rural areas, where there is no public transportation, or in suburban areas where the residential sections were designed with the assumption that everyone drives automobiles. Even in urban areas, older adults who cannot drive find themselves isolated.

- *Nutritional services*—Nutritional services may be home delivered (meals-on-wheels) or served in a group setting. Meals-on-wheels serves elderly, disabled, or at-risk persons identified by social service agencies or even by concerned neighbors. Usually the service delivers a meal in the middle of the day to be reheated at the client's convenience. Often a sandwich and side dishes are added to ensure two balanced, nutritious meals per day. Dining in a group setting (called "congregate dining") offers social benefits as well as nutrition. Sites may be schools, senior centers, or churches. These sites frequently offer additional services, such as health promotion, financial and insurance counseling, and recreation.

In response to public concerns about the quality of nursing facilities, the care they provide, and their adherence to governmental regulations, and also to meet the needs of residents who faced problems in their nursing homes, the ombudsman program was created in 1972 by the Public Health Service. The program was transferred to the Administration on Aging in 1974, and in 1978 Congress mandated that each state develop a long-term care ombudsman program. The function of the ombudsman is to resolve problems on behalf of residents in order to improve their overall well-being. The ombudsman's role combines active advocacy and representation of residents' interests through a variety of activities:

- Advocate for policy change when indicated
- Evaluate laws and regulations
- Provide education to the public and to the facility staff
- Distribute program data
- Promote the development of resident and family councils

Interventions take place in the nursing home or board-and-care facility where the older adult resides.

As managed-care organizations have increased their services and influence, applying cost containment strategies to decisions about who may qualify for placement in a long-term care facility, the demand for ombudsman services has grown. Increasingly, the ombudsman's services are provided in clients' homes and in community-based settings, since many technologically advanced procedures have been transferred from hospitals and nursing homes to home settings. (See Chapter 8 for more information on ombudsman programs, including how to contact a local ombudsman.)

# 2

# Theories of the Aging Process

AGING IS A familiar process, taking place in living things all around us. Yet we are only beginning to understand what happens as we grow older. There are over 300 plausible theories that explain the clusters of physical and psychological signs of aging. The reason there are so many is that the study of biologic gerontology is a relatively recent discipline with less than twenty years of funded research. Even with expanded research, it's likely that a single umbrella theory would be inadequate because the many aging processes would be very difficult to mesh under one theory. Most of the varied theories originate from studying the action of aging changes that accumulate over time.

While no single theory accounts for all of the observations about aging, recent research suggests that the reason people age is under genetic control with some contributions from environmental factors. Significantly, current theories describe aging events either as occurring randomly and accumulating with time (stochastic) or as being predetermined (nonstochastic). Either way, these theories of aging may use a biologic or a psychosocial perspective.

# The Biology of Aging

As we age, the most obvious changes include the changes to our bodies. Although the difference between normal aging and disease may seem negligible, aging has some characteristics that distinguish it from disease:

- The aging process damages organisms and reduces function.
- The change is gradual and progressive.
- The aging process is intrinsic and not affected by modifying environmental factors.
- The alteration is universal, meaning it affects all members of the species.

Of course, there are individual differences in the rates of biologic aging. We can easily observe two seventy-year-old men and find one with many more youthful qualities than the other. As a result, scientists have concluded that people age biologically at different rates. The changes brought about by aging begin in different parts of the body at different times, and the rate of annual change varies among various cells, tissues, and organs, as well as from person to person. Biologic aging, sometimes called functional aging, is difficult to measure. Knowing biologic age would be much more informative than knowing chronological age, but as yet there is no precise way of measuring biologic age. The most widely used biologic theories of aging are genetic programming theory, immunity theory, stress theory, error theory, and mutation theory.

## *Genetic Programming*

According to the *genetic programming theory*, a person's life span is programmed at birth through genes or is the result of changes in genetic material, DNA, that occur with age.

During the late 1950s, Leonard Hayflick and Paul Moorehead began studying the effects of cancer-causing viruses on normal cells in culture. In maintaining such cultures, they observed that cells experienced a limited number of divisions and then died. In 1961 Hayflick and Moorehead noted that human fetal fibroblastic cells underwent an average of fifty divisions in laboratory experiments before losing the ability to replicate themselves. They proposed that aging is intrinsic to the cell and not solely dependent on outside influences.

The initial premise of the genetic programming theory, sometimes referred to as the biologic or genetic clock theory, begins with the idea that the body begins with a base of genetic information that is distributed in an orderly manner. As time passes, cells undergo development, maturation, and cessation of activity. Evidence of these changes includes graying of hair, beginning of menopause, wrinkling of skin, and numerous other changes that are considered normal parts of aging, not symptoms of disease.

However, there have been some successful research efforts to genetically alter an individual cell's aging schedule. Researchers have isolated a gene, MORF4, which when mutated appears to turn off the aging program in some cultured human cells, allowing them to divide indefinitely. Nevertheless, it is probable that most human cells never reach their potential limit of divisions. Therefore, it is extremely unlikely that the cellular aging process is solely responsible for the signs of aging. Further experiments have supported a variety of other mechanisms.

## Immunity Theory

The basis for *immunity theory* is the possibility that the way autoimmune disease advances is related to the aging process. As cells of the immune system age, they become less uniform and more irregular in the way they behave. In some cases these immune system cells identify normal body cells as foreign or abnormal and they attack these targets.

Research into immune theories provides insight into many health problems experienced by older adults, such as cancer, diabetes, dementia, and certain vascular diseases.

## Stress Theory

The *stress theory* is very familiar to the layperson as well as the health practitioner because the effects of stress on physical and psychological health have been widely discussed and documented. Stresses to the body can cause damage and lead to conditions such as gastric ulcers, heart attacks, and thyroiditis. The physical changes are real and arise from basic changes in the body's cells, tissue, and organs. The basic cellular metabolic rate decreases, and cellular division and growth are limited. Like a complicated machine, the body functions less efficiently with prolonged use. However, the rate of this decrement in function varies greatly from individual to individual.

Differences in the way individuals react to life's stresses limit the applicability of this theory. One person may be overwhelmed by a moderately busy schedule, whereas another may become uncomfortable when faced with a slow, dull pace. There are those who are stimulated by stressful, demanding situations and who have developed strategies not only for managing stress but also for improving skills in assessing situations and prioritizing actions. Even accepting the fact that wear and tear on the body, such as physical stress, will cause the body to age and gradually wear out from use over the years, the rate at which this occurs is highly individualized.

## Error Theory

Underlying the *error theory* is the premise that nothing works perfectly forever and that there are no guaranteed repair processes. This may explain why formerly "perfect" systems age and fail.

Advocates of the error theory argue that faults in various molecules accumulate to a point where metabolic failures occur, resulting in age changes and, finally, death. On the surface, this is a compelling theory. There is indisputable evidence that errors do occur and that, although repair processes exist, they are not perfect and do not function indefinitely. The error theory can be traced to an earlier hypothesis, that gene mutations might produce age changes.

## Mutation Theory

According to the *mutation theory*, gene mutations might produce age changes. Mutations are random events, errors that occur in the genetic apparatus of cells. When mutations occur in the genes of a sperm or egg (the *germ cells*), the offspring of the sperm or egg will differ somewhat from the parents. Natural selection may then either favor the change, permitting it to be passed on to that animal's progeny, or reject the change, in which case the animal will die or fail to achieve reproductive success. If the mutations instead occur in the *somatic cells* (cells that are not germ cells), the mutation theory of aging says the mutations could result in aging.

Little evidence exists to support the mutation and error theories, however. The popularity of these theories, which was quite high a decade or two ago, has therefore declined significantly in recent years.

Each of the theories offering clues to aging raises many questions. For example, many of the symptoms that are attributed to poor circulation in the elderly may actually be the effects of the death of nondividing cells. Metabolic rate, genetic background, diet, and environmental factors affect the frequent alterations in the aging body.

# How Long Can We Hope to Live?

The biology of aging involves two measures that might sound the same but have quite different meanings: life expectancy and life span. *Life expectancy* is a statistical measurement about the members of a group; it represents the average length of life of a person within that group. In contrast, *life span* defines the maximum limit of human life, the age beyond which no one can expect to live. The figure that is currently acceptable among scientists is about 115 years. Thus, if you are a fifty-year-old white female, you have a life expectancy of thirty-three more years. This is an average, so some white females will live longer or shorter lives, but probably none will live beyond the human life span of 115.

Improved health practices, advances in pharmacology, and new technologies have continued to increase life expectancy, but it is unlikely that life span will increase markedly. Nevertheless, some people advocate prolongevity, the significant extension of the length of life. These advocates offer examples of exceptionally long-lived populations in remote Andean and Russian mountain villages, where residents have claimed ages of 120, 130, and older. They have offered some explanations for this phenomenon:

- The natural environment was pristine. The air, water, and plants were uncontaminated.
- Diet was ideal. The villagers ate very little meat, and what they did eat was low in fat.
- Life in the mountainous terrain demanded constant physical exertion, which benefited their hearts and lungs.

However, the claims of the "super aged" are doubtful because of lack of documentation, incomplete record keeping, or outright exaggeration.

Still, we can learn from the investigation of these groups. These people have common factors that may contribute to overall longer life expectancy. One is their exemplary dietary practices, including high intake of vegetables and fiber and low intake of calories. Members of these groups get regular exercise. A final factor may be sociability. The groups studied were friendly and gregarious.

# The Psychology and Sociology of Aging

Along with changes in their bodies, older adults experience psychological and social changes. These changes happen in concert and they have a significant impact on each other. Based on observing these changes, social scientists have developed three prominent psychosocial theories of aging: disengagement theory, activity theory, and continuity theory.

## *Disengagement Theory*

Some psychologists have noticed a tendency of elderly people to spend more time alone, reflecting on their past. This led psychologists John Cumming and Mary Henry to propose the *disengagement theory*. This theory is as controversial today as when it was first proposed in 1961.

According to the theory, a mutual withdrawal or disengagement results in decreased interaction between the aging person and others in the social system to which the person belongs, which coincides with the older adult's lessened capabilities and diminished interest in "younger" activities. The supposed benefit to older individuals is that they can then reflect and focus on themselves (since they are freed from former societal roles). This time is then spent largely in isolation (often marked by moving into a retirement or nursing home) reviewing one's life, and preparing for the ultimate disengagement—death.

It is important to remember that in the 1960s, when this theory was proposed, the typical way of life for the elderly may have influenced social scientists' perception of what was possible or optimal. The foundation of the theory made sense at a time when there was a shorter life expectancy, an earlier onset of disability, physically demanding work roles, mandatory retirement, and few organized activities for older adults.

Despite the initial logic, it is easy to see the negative aspects of the disengagement theory. It seems to describe elderly persons as incompetent and old age as a time of sitting around, waiting to die. In addition, encouraging an older adult to move into a completely different housing setting seems to be an ineffective way to strengthen the roles and activities of the elderly. Since the disengagement theory was formulated at a time when society defined separate roles for men and women, another weakness within the theory is that it is based on the distinctive pattern of engagement for men without considering the changing role of women.

Many current gerontological researchers and practitioners oppose the implications of this theory because it moves older people into an area of physical or social separation. Particularly disturbing is the implication that the elderly are automatically incompetent and should no longer be involved in the societal roles they once filled. Gerontologists further dispute the perception of old age as a waiting period for death.

Instead, current theories embrace the idea that positive experiences can be had outside a group setting through continued interaction with the population at large. When older adults do choose group settings, senior centers, assisted-living communities, and congregate living can provide opportunities for them to continue their active lives through influential voting blocs, expanded social opportunities, the development of new skills, and other enriching activities.

## Activity Theory

The *activity theory* proposes that people age most successfully when they participate fully in daily activities. This theory proposes that there is a positive relationship between activity and satisfaction in life. If individuals are able to maintain activities established in the middle years of life, the adjustment to later life will be agreeable.

This theory considers aging to be a time of change and loss. The many physical changes that accompany normal aging, and the associated disease processes, often result in physical and cognitive impairments in varying degrees. The losses are functional, intellectual, and psychological, arising from these initial impairments. Coinciding with these losses is the transition from work-related positions of value (for example, manager, professor, or doctor) to the less-valued role of retiree. The departure from the primary role conferred by belonging to the workforce to the generic role of retiree demands an adaptation, and people make that change with varying degrees of success. At the same time, people in this stage of life experience losses from the deaths of relatives, friends, and other loved ones.

The entrance into extended leisure is a high predictor of life satisfaction. Social interaction, development of new skills, and the maximizing of growth experiences distinguish a positive adaptation to this period. Leisure can foster well-being by enhancing self-esteem and improving the individual's sense of mental and physical competence. It also permits the individual to exercise some control over his or her environment. Leisure provides opportunities for personal growth and accomplishment. The failure to maximize leisure opportunities results in deficiencies in these areas. Unsuccessful aging occurs if a person disengages from formerly enjoyed activities, becomes socially isolated, and experiences physical and cognitive decline.

The activity theory suggests that older adults age successfully when they maintain a comfortable, satisfactory activity level. This consists of enjoying and expanding old pastimes, learning new skills, developing social contacts, and remaining physically active. Its proponents believe that people who maintain normal actions and social roles (both formal and informal) and engage in solitary as well as social pursuits are more likely to enjoy enhanced self-esteem and life satisfaction. If the activities of older adults are in social settings conducive to developing relationships, they reinforce positive self-concepts and enjoy greater satisfaction with their lives. Less successful adaptation to aging resembles aging according to the disengagement theory; the person exhibits lack of interest in previously enjoyed activities and relationships.

Studies have found that contentment with life, volunteerism, and feelings of usefulness are interdependent. The research indicates that social activity has a productive purpose and can be used as an intervention to foster life satisfaction and successful aging. The widely held assumption that retirement is synonymous with radical changes in lifestyle and productivity is often mistaken. Research supports the finding that the elderly generally maintain activity levels similar to those of their middle years.

Older adults do make changes in the specific activities they participate in, because of the move from full- or part-time employment to retirement. These activities may be intrinsically pleasurable, or they may meet more demanding cognitive or psychosocial needs.

## Continuity Theory

According to the *continuity theory*, the people who age most successfully are those who extend the habits, preferences, lifestyles, and relationships of midlife into late life. Scientific investigation has indicated that variables measured in midlife are strong predictors of outcomes in later life. Many psychological and social characteristics are stable throughout a person's lifetime.

Generally, late life does not represent a radical break with the past. Changes often occur gradually and even imperceptibly. Most people skirt the potholes in the road of life by using their well-honed coping skills. Past experiences, decisions, and behaviors form the basis for present and future decisions and behaviors.

The foundation of the continuity theory is that as middle-aged and elderly adults experience age-related changes, they rely more and more on existing resources. Continuity is the subjective perception that changes associated with aging are linked to an individual's personality. It does not mean that people will successfully adjust to changes in their lives. Rather, it proposes that as people contend with the changes in their lives, they use existing resources and coping strategies.

Continuity theory allows and even encourages change within the older person's life. Dynamic changes in continuity do not fundamentally change the unique characteristics of the individual; rather, they allow an individual to adapt to age-related life changes.

Older adults cultivate *internal continuity* by using their experience, emotions, coping mechanisms, and problem solving skills to manage late life changes. People generally strive for *external continuity* by becoming involved with familiar activities, environments, and people. These strategies are a practical way to cope with the physical and mental changes associated with normal aging.

The continuity theory describes continuity as a practiced response to life situations. Growing old does not require broad, sweeping changes in beliefs, interests, or preferences, even though a person inevitably experiences traumatic changes such as serious illness, death of a spouse, or an unplanned move. In fact, research on a major life disruption, stroke, and the attempts of stroke patients to adapt gave another dimension to the continuity theory—the adaptation to illness. According to the research, elderly stroke patients employed internal and external strategies to reestablish continuity in their lives. For example, they employed the internal strategy of prayer and the external strategy of interaction with family members.

Five age-related factors which affected the patient's response to the sudden change from good health to stroke recovery are diminished stamina, lack of social support, financial constraints, other recent losses, more than one chronic illness. These factors often intensify the challenge to recover from a stroke (or other sudden, debilitating accident or illness). At times, these challenges can pose barriers that patients regard as insurmountable. Continuity theory is both enhanced and expanded when patient's reactions to this type of situation are studied.

So far, research has provided support for the continuity theory. However, further studies are needed to answer some remaining questions:

- How do individuals experience discontinuity caused by the onset of chronic illness late in life?
- Do efforts to maintain continuity despite late-onset chronic illness differ from efforts made at younger ages?
- What variables differentiate the discontinuity experienced by elderly adults from that experienced by younger persons?

From observing the ways elders maintain continuity during disruptive life events, clinicians can develop helpful, holistic interventions. Besides these formal interventions, the elderly and their caregivers can enhance the adjustment to aging by maintaining activities and social supports that help keep up past lifestyles over which the elderly have some control.

The continuity theory is also referred to as the developmental theory, because it compares factors of personality and behavior in old age to similar factors during other phases of the life cycle. Healthy psychosocial characteristics evolve as a consequence of successfully completing developmental tasks—those challenging experiences that elders (and others) must meet and manage. Concepts and patterns developed over a lifetime will determine whether individuals remain engaged and active or become remote and apathetic. Therefore, barring unusual circumstances—for example, dementia or drug side effects—personality and basic patterns of behavior remain virtually unchanged as individuals age.

The view of aging as an ongoing developmental process affords older adults a range of opportunities to gain a new sense of satisfaction. The unique features of each individual allow for multiple adaptations to aging. The potential for a variety of reactions gives this theory credibility.

# Successful Aging

Advances in medicine, research, and social systems have made it possible to help the elderly acquire useful information in order to age successfully. Research shows that the elderly are living longer and healthier lives. The aging body is capable of adapting to changes in lifestyles, and more important, the aging brain is capable of processing significant amounts of new information. Granted, learning occurs in different ways, and it occurs more slowly in the elderly than in younger adults, but the myth "You can't teach an old dog new tricks" has been debunked.

Clearly, aging has a genetic influence. Even so, about 70 percent of changes in the heart, liver, and kidneys experienced by the aging person are the result of choices individuals make during their lives. About 50 percent of the changes in the aging brain are related to lifestyle. Older adults can take steps to maintain physical and cognitive function. For example, exercising, abstaining from smoking, and practicing appropriate dietary habits contribute to successful physical aging. Remaining active and engaged mentally supports cognitive function. Practicing these behaviors empowers the elderly.

In the 4,000 years before 1900, human life expectancy increased about twenty-seven years. From 1900 to 1990, it increased another twenty-seven to thirty years. Currently, with the gradual reduction in the mortality rates in infancy, youth, and middle age, and more recently in late life, average life expectancy of women aged sixty-five has been extended fifteen years; in men, about eight years. The majority of people born in the United States live well past retirement. As described in Chapter 1, the age structure of our population has changed dramatically.

Disability rates in older people have declined in the United States over the past several decades, including in people over the age of eighty-five. The percentage of older persons living in nursing homes has also declined and is now 5.2 percent for adults over the age of sixty-five. While at one time people worried that morbidity (the rate of illness) would expand as a result of the increase in longevity, the data suggest that morbidity has shrunk. This means that with better disease prevention and treatment, the period between the onset of severe disability and death is compressed into fewer years. The majority of elderly adults are not necessarily ill, as once was feared.

Gerontological research, formerly preoccupied with disease, diagnosis, medication, and nursing home admission, now emphasizes the age-related nonpathologic changes, rather than disease-related changes that impair function. The focus is no longer on the negative aspects of aging, but on more studies of health maintenance and prevention of disease, as well as why the elderly are managing as well as they are.

Obviously, avoiding disease and disability is an essential component of successful aging. However, additional, critical issues have emerged—namely, the maintenance of high cognitive and physical function. Older adults age successfully if they are engaged with life, have a strong social support system, and are involved in productive activities. Therefore, remaining healthy and active increases the ability to maximize cognitive and physical function.

## Normal Aging or "Usual" Aging?

In the elderly population compared to younger Americans, there is an increase in blood sugar, waist-hip ratio, insulin level, blood pressure, and blood homocystine. These measurements are all associated with present and future health. When these measures are above normal limits, diseases such as diabetes mellitus and hypertension are likely.

An aged person who is not diseased is referred to as "normal." But using the word *normal* to describe the health status of an older adult can be misleading. The term implies that the person is less likely to develop a health problem than someone whose status is not "normal." But if disease-related measures like blood sugar and blood pressure are elevated, even within the range typically experienced by others of the same age, the person may be at risk for health problems. Under these circumstances, a more accurate term than *normal aging* would be *usual aging*.

In the "usual" aging population, blood pressure is rising, and so are the associated risks. Elevated blood pressure is a risk factor for stroke and for cardiovascular events. The higher it is, the greater the risk for morbidity and mortality.

Two components define usual aging: intrinsic factors and extrinsic factors. Genetics, an intrinsic factor, strongly influences aging. However, important noninheritable, extrinsic characteristics, including environment and lifestyle, are just as threatening. For example, the percentage of high-density lipoproteins (HDL), or "good" cholesterol, found in serum lipids declines slightly with advancing age, regardless of a strong genetic background. A person can have great genes, but if elevated LDL ("bad" cholesterol) and lowered HDL levels are ignored, good genes will not be able to help. Analyses of lung function, body weight, waist-hip ratio, and blood pressure clearly indicate that successful aging is much more than choosing parents wisely. Since people have control over extrinsic factors (such as weight), they can affect many intrinsic factors (such as blood pressure). Older adults are largely responsible for their own old-age situations.

While usual aging has risks, people can modify these risks. For example, a study published in 1995 reported that participants lowered a variety of risk factors. These individuals had high waist-hip ratio, obesity, hypertension, and a tendency toward hyperglycemia (elevated blood sugar levels) and hyperinsulinemia (excessive insulin in the bloodstream). They lowered these risk factors over a nine-month period on a medically supervised weight reduction program.

As mentioned earlier, successful aging also depends on maintaining high cognitive functioning. To identify factors that predict the maintenance of high cognitive function, researchers studied verbal and nonverbal memory, language, conceptualization, and visual and spatial ability in a group of well elderly. The researchers found that the maintenance of high cognitive function, as measured by these factors in these healthy elders, depended on their education, peak pulmonary flow rate (a measure of lung function), strenuous activity, and a sense of self-efficacy.

As in this study, challenging physical activity and cognitive function are interrelated. Increased physical activity influences the chemical substances that promote new brain cells. Exercise also increases blood flow, which delivers more oxygen to the brain, thus improving brain function.

Aging well requires that the older adult take certain constructive steps to ensure health and well-being:

- Improve diet and activity, which affect physical health and the ability to perform tasks of daily living.
- Increase exercise, which plays a valuable part in maintaining physical function.
- Cultivate social supports, such as family and friends.
- Use the mechanics of mental functioning to cope with the cognitive changes in old age, using purposeful activity to maintain identity and foster well-being.

**Table 2.1 Measures That Help People Age Successfully**

| Activity | How It Helps |
|---|---|
| Engaging in challenging physical activity | Brisk walks increase blood flow to all body systems, including the brain. |
| Balancing activity and leisure | A good balance helps to define nonwork time. |
| Building self-esteem | High self-esteem improves performance and problem solving. |
| Expanding social contacts | Involvement with others lessens risk of depression and provides intellectual stimulation. |
| Improving flexibility | A flexible person adapts activities or seeks substitutes that meet social, intellectual, or leisure needs. |

Table 2.1 summarizes some commonly accepted principles for aging successfully.

# Ethnic Barriers to Successful Aging

As we saw in Chapter 1, the experience of being elderly in America differs somewhat among racial and cultural groups. Some of these differences present barriers to aging successfully.

## *African Americans*

Education levels and health status are significant markers in diminishing cognitive processes once considered inevitable outcomes of old age. Research has shown a relationship between higher educational levels, healthy lifestyles, and unimpaired cognition. According to the research, the lower the educational level, the poorer the health status, and thus a greater probability for cognitive impairment. Few studies of this relationship have focused specifically on African-Americans, yet identifying factors for maintenance, decline, or enhancement of cognitive functioning that are prevalent in African-Americans contributes to the understanding of cognitive aging for all elderly.

In one study of cognitive functioning, conducted in 1997, 224 successfully aging African-Americans aged seventy to eighty years old were tracked for two years to identify risk factors. The researchers found that decline in cognitive function was not an inevitable result of advancing age. Nearly half the sample interviewed improved or maintained their level of cognitive performance over the two-year tracking period. The findings of the study showed some factors associated with cognitive improvement or decline:

- People who rated themselves as healthy were significantly more likely to show an improvement in cognitive functioning.
- People who experienced poor performance on a common lung function test were more likely to suffer cognitive decline.
- People with lower education levels tended to experience a greater decline.

In one case, a group of elderly African-Americans born and raised with limited opportunities, particularly in education, health care, housing, and employment managed to exhibit a high degree of strength and resiliency. Members of this group have successfully managed the problems and frustrations of old age for several reasons:

- *Frequent and regular voting practices*—According to analysis of political participation among elderly African-Americans, we know that this group, as a whole, is more likely to vote than its younger counterparts, especially in the case of those who attend church regularly. The positive relationship between church attendance and voting behavior suggests that churches may be a critical element in political mobilization within black communities.
- *Strong kinship bonds*—Intergenerational relationships are significant among African-Americans. Traditionally, the family structure involves three generations. Grandparents frequently

see their role as passing on traditions and culture. In addition, grandparents may act as surrogates when parents work, are disabled, or are unavailable. However, cultural values associated with caring for aged family members are being affected by demographic trends on a national level. Declining birthrates, decreasing rates of marriage, increased divorce, and substance abuse limit the number of persons available to provide care and assistance to the growing numbers of older family members.

- *High level of participation in religion*—The church often occupies a central role, providing support within minority communities. It also offers a mutual aid system to extend economic, emotional, and spiritual assistance, as well as opportunities for African-American elders to perform meaningful roles that are valued by their community.

## Hispanic Americans

Hispanic Americans are the fastest-growing minority population in the United States. Although they share a common language, this group represents several subgroups, including Mexican-Americans, Puerto Ricans, Cubans, and Latin Americans. Hispanic Americans enjoy the close-knit familial bonds and the participation in religion that African-Americans do, but they also experience many barriers to successful aging in the areas of finance, housing, and health.

U.S. Hispanics have been undereducated and underemployed for many years. Consequently, they are poorly prepared, as a group, to meet their financial needs in old age, and they experience high rates of poverty. They also are more likely to be unemployed than African-American or white older adults are. Many are unprepared to support themselves independently, and they rely totally on supplemental income derived from Social Security and other government assistance such as food stamps, Medicaid, and fuel assistance.

Housing for Hispanic elderly tends to be in economically depressed areas, yet these settings are familiar to them. Elderly Hispanics in this situation know their neighbors and derive a sense of security from them. However, living in high-crime areas places them at risk. Also, the location of these neighborhoods is not always convenient to the many services the older adults require, such as medical clinics, Social Security offices, and supermarkets and drugstores.

Physical health is a major issue for Hispanic elderly. Of all groups of adults aged sixty-five and over, a larger number of Hispanics have at least one chronic illness and some limitations in activities of daily living. Diabetes, hypertension, and cancer are prevalent in this community of older adults.

## Asian Americans

The myth of the "model minority" often applied to Asian-Americans not only conceals economic disparities and ethnic differences, it may increase tensions between the Asian community and other minority groups. In fact, elderly Asians face their share of obstacles to successful aging:

- The false perception that access to social services is readily available
- Rapid changes in family structure and traditions
- The complicated health care system

Asian-American populations are statistically small, and there has been little funding for social services to meet their specific needs. Compounding the situation is the great diversity in language, cultural background, socioeconomic status, and health status existing among the various Asian groups.

The aging Asian-American population is predominantly female. The increased participation of Asian women in the workforce disrupts the tradition of women caring for the elderly at home. In the past, high birthrates and lower levels of life expectancy ensured that the small numbers of Asian elderly were cared for by ample numbers of children and grandchildren. However, family structure and function have changed significantly.

The convoluted U.S. health care system has become increasingly bewildering following the trend to privatization accompanied by changes in market strategies. Asian-Americans have a high rate of non-compliance with Western prescriptions, usually relying instead on traditional health practices. Moreover, inadequate budget appropriation for services, language problems, and perceived anti-immigrant treatment by Western health care providers have increased the isolation of elderly Asian-Americans from available health care services.

## Success Stories

Historically, humans have lived an agricultural existence. Life expectancy was short, and the concept of retirement was unknown. The few who did live long usually controlled the family and were held in high status in the community. Other old-age survivors were revered elders in their religious-ethnic communities. In contrast, the urban realities of the twentieth century and beyond reveal a great number of older adults well past seventy and an increase in the number of retired persons. This population includes many encouraging examples of adults who have aged successfully.

In a unique study of elderly Israeli professionals, Benjamin Chetkow-Yanoov, DSW, a social work researcher, examined a group of older adults, who, in spite of being afflicted with many of the common limitations of old age, aged successfully. These elders made use of healthy coping skills in order to manage their late-life crises, such as increasing frailty, deaths of friends and family members, and retirement.

The study drew participants from seven professions: social workers, nurses, educators, artists, biochemists, politicians, and bureaucrats. Within these seven professions, the researchers found four distinct types of leaders:

1. Individually active persons who concentrated on study and personal hobbies, rated reading as very important to their intellectual stimulation, and were often called on to give lectures related to their disciplines
2. Socially active persons who enjoyed club activities, assisted their neighbors, and rated helping others as high among their priorities

3. Organizational leaders who served on boards and commit-
   tees, engaged in public relations, and helped raise funds
4. Community leaders who were politically active, served on
   public commissions, had their writings published, and
   received public recognition for their leadership

Although the elderly adults in this group were not dependent on
family members, did not participate in welfare, and were not confined
to institutions, they did have to face the same late-life crises as elders
in any other comparable group. In spite of these drawbacks, they found
fulfillment within the urban society during their advancing years.

The researchers looked for characteristics of group members that
might shed light on why they aged successfully. Characteristics shared
by group members included raised expectations and high levels of functional competence, which challenged the stereotypes and policies of
public social services, which concentrates on the frail aged. In addition, members of the group had five other characteristics in common:

1. High educational performance
2. A perception that their own health was good
3. Enjoyment of their preretirement work
4. An optimistic view of life in general and of the future in
   particular
5. A continued association with a wide range and number of
   social contacts

Members of the group studied also shared a desire to remain
active, as well as beliefs that they had some influence over life events
and that change was a necessary stimulus for growth.

The outcome confirmed the study's hypothesis, which was that the
problems of aging are not insurmountable. The elderly professionals
used their skills to remain active throughout their "third age." They
did not "retire from" anything. Rather, they entered new fields for
which they had not had time in the past, or they practiced their skills
in a variety of new volunteer settings.

# 3

# Nutrition, Aging, and Older Adults

AT ONE TIME, most people thought the nutritional requirements of younger and older adults were essentially the same. However, as the number and influence of older adults has grown, research on the importance of nutrition for the elderly has increased. Such nutrition research identifies the important essential nutrients governing tissue repair and resistance to infection, and demonstrates how older adults can take advantage of such findings.

Scientific studies clearly have shown that lifestyle choices play even more of a role than heredity in deciding the level of health and function in a person's later years. Good nutrition profoundly influences health, quality of life, and longevity. Furthermore, it is the foundation for maintaining cognitive and physical function. Unhealthful eating and a sedentary lifestyle contribute to 14 percent of preventable deaths each year, a figure exceeded only by tobacco use.

Elderly people are less physically active than younger adults are. Consequently, their energy requirements decrease, as do their caloric needs. Adults over the age of seventy-five need about 80 percent of the calories required for a younger adult. However, more than one-fourth of older men and over one-third of elderly women are consuming more than that. As a result, they are obese.

Weight increases slowly during the aging process. Men reach a peak in their fifties, and women in their seventies. After that, a person's weight begins to decrease very slowly. But this pattern can be deceptive. As they accumulate adipose (fat) tissue, men and women lose lean body tissue. It is to the advantage of all adults to minimize this shift and control the unfavorable increase in weight by achieving a balance between diet and exercise.

People who ignore the importance of obesity control risk an increase in illnesses and earlier death. Among the diseases linked directly to the excessive accumulation of fatty tissue are diabetes, hypertension, coronary artery disease, and cancer.

# Building Blocks of Nutrition

Good nutrition involves eating and drinking enough of the substances the body needs for energy and good health. Among the basics of good nutrition are organic compounds called *macronutrients*. There are three kinds of macronutrients: protein, fats, and carbohydrates. In addition, the body needs *micronutrients* in the form of vitamins and minerals, as well as plenty of water.

## *Macronutrients*

*Protein* is a vital substance that controls most of the structural processes of the body. Recent research indicates that elderly adults have a slightly increased need for this nutrient. Many elderly who have had hip fractures, pressure sores, and impaired wound healing are not eating enough protein. Conversely, older adults who consume adequate protein have greater recovery rates and fewer complications from acute and chronic illnesses. Protein is present in meat, fish, poultry, eggs, and cheese, as well as certain plant sources. An older adult should consume about 15 percent of calories, or the equivalent of two glasses of low-fat milk plus one meat portion (based on the USDA recommended portion), each day to meet protein demands.

*Carbohydrates* are key sources of energy for the body. However, excessive consumption of refined carbohydrates is equivalent to ingesting too much fat and too many calories. Complex carbohydrates are superior because the number of calories per unit of food is lower and the concentration of nutrients is higher. Furthermore, fiber is a component of complex carbohydrates, and this substance is extremely important to optimal gastrointestinal function. Complex carbohydrates and rich stores of fiber are in fruits, vegetables, whole-grain cereals, whole-grain bread, and pasta. Older adults should get more than 50 percent of their daily caloric intake from complex carbohydrates.

*Fats* provide energy and help to distribute vitamins A, D, E, and K. In addition, fat improves the taste of certain foods and increases our feeling of satiety. However, people of all ages should use fats and oils sparingly. In the average U.S. diet, about 40 percent of the total calories come from fat, whereas the recommended intake is no more than about 30 percent. Excessive consumption of fat contributes directly to atherosclerosis. In the industrialized world, the arterial damage caused by atherosclerosis is related to half of the death rate.

## Micronutrients

Other components of good nutrition are the micronutrients, the vitamins and minerals in food. These substances are often lacking in the diets of the elderly. Minerals are especially important, because they enable the body to carry on normal chemical processes. Most minerals are readily supplied in food, with the exceptions of calcium and iron. Therefore, calcium and iron supplements are essential to optimize diets of the elderly. However, to remedy any deficiencies safely, elderly individuals should have a professional evaluation of their calcium and iron intake. This precaution is important because as people age, their metabolism and organ function decrease, making mineral supplementation potentially toxic.

## Water

Although the human body can survive several weeks without food, it probably cannot survive more than one week without water. Water is essential to life for several reasons. Most basically, it provides vital support for all internal chemical reactions. The urinary system in particular depends on water for its function. Also, insufficient water is a common cause of constipation.

The fluid requirement of older adults is a minimum of six to eight glasses of water daily. Less fluid intake contributes to the development of dehydration, a risk encountered by many elderly persons.

Often elderly persons deliberately restrict their fluid intake because they fear episodes of incontinence. They may take their medications with barely enough water to swallow a pill or capsule. This behavior can cause adverse drug effects, and swallowing some capsules without adequate water can damage the esophagus.

In long-term care where evening meals are usually served in the late afternoon, many hours elapse between dinner and the next day's breakfast. Fluids should be offered during the evening to prevent dehydration from developing overnight.

# Age-Related Digestive Changes

Ensuring that older adults eat enough of the right foods to balance their health and energy needs can be a challenge for clinicians and caregivers. The complex physiological changes and the psychosocial aspects of aging markedly affect the nutritional requirements of the elderly. The table details age-related changes that occur in some organs of the digestive tract, as well as the way these affect the ability to digest and obtain nutrients.

# Ingredients of a Healthful Diet

The cornerstone of a diet containing essential nutrients is the Recommended Dietary Allowance (RDA) guidelines established by the Food and Nutrition Board of the National Academy of Sciences. The RDAs, first established to ensure that the servicemen of World War II were properly nourished, are an intricate guide for optimizing health. However, for calculating the nutrients required by the elderly, the RDAs have limitations:

- The RDAs are aimed at preventing nutritional deficiency, not preventing disease, so they may understate optimal amounts of nutrients.

### Table 3.1 Age-Related Changes in the Digestive System

| Organ | Age-Related Change | Functional Change |
|---|---|---|
| Esophagus | Reduced peristaltic action; delay in emptying | Gastroesophageal reflux |
| Salivary glands | Decreased saliva flow | Dry mouth |
| Stomach | Decreased secretion of digestive acid; poor absorption of iron | Iron-deficiency anemia |
| Intestines | Reduced peristaltic action | Constipation; flatulence; diverticulosis |
| Liver | Decrease in size | Reduced ability to synthesize protein; reduced ability to metabolize drugs |
| Senses of taste, smell | Decrease in number of taste buds; decrease in nerve endings for smell | Less appetite; less pleasure in eating |

- They are recommendations for healthy population groups.
- In setting the RDA levels, the board did not consider diet-drug and food-nutrient interactions.
- To set RDAs for the elderly, the board simply extrapolated from studies of the younger population.

The U.S. Department of Agriculture (USDA) simplified the complex RDA standards by developing the Food Guide Pyramid, a visual display that is easy to read and is therefore more informative than the numerical guidelines (Figure 3.1). It is a general guide, an outline, of what to eat, based on dietary guidelines. The Food Guide Pyramid is reprinted here, and the USDA offers a free, detailed description of it (phone 1-800-222-2225 and request publication number NIH 99-4258).

To adapt these guidelines to the needs of the elderly, researchers at Tufts University developed a modified Food Guide Pyramid for adults over seventy years old. This model resembles the USDA's original food pyramid but more accurately reflects the dietary needs of older adults.

## Figure 3.1 The Food Guide Pyramid

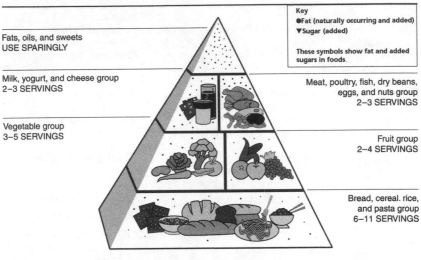

Source: U.S. Department of Agriculture, Department of Health and Human Services.

The modified pyramid, shown in Figure 3.2, recognizes the significance of an elderly person's reduced energy needs. Because elderly people need fewer calories, the nutritional value of each calorie is especially important. That principle is the basis for key differences in the adjusted food pyramid:

- The modified pyramid indicates nutrient-dense choices in all food categories.
- It stresses the importance of fiber and adequate hydration.
- It suggests the possible need for dietary supplements—namely, calcium and vitamin D to improve bone health and vitamin $B_{12}$ to optimize nerve function.

Ideally, an elderly person's diet should be low in saturated fatty acids and cholesterol; low in sugar, salt, and alcohol; and high in vegetables, fruits, and whole-grain products. Dairy products should be primarily low-fat foods. For individuals with a lactose incompatibility, a growing selection of lactose-free foods enables elderly adults to consume the important foods in this group. When selecting from the meat,

## Figure 3.2  Modified Food Guide Pyramid for Adults over Seventy Years

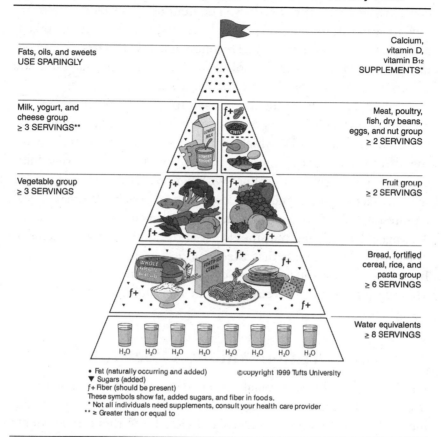

Fats, oils, and sweets
USE SPARINGLY

Calcium,
vitamin D,
vitamin B₁₂
SUPPLEMENTS*

Milk, yogurt, and
cheese group
≥ 3 SERVINGS**

Meat, poultry,
fish, dry beans,
eggs, and nut group
≥ 2 SERVINGS

Vegetable group
≥ 3 SERVINGS

Fruit group
≥ 2 SERVINGS

Bread, fortified
cereal, rice, and
pasta group
≥ 6 SERVINGS

Water equivalents
≥ 8 SERVINGS

• Fat (naturally occurring and added)          ©copyright 1999 Tufts University
▼ Sugars (added)
ƒ+ Fiber (should be present)
These symbols show fat, added sugars, and fiber in foods.
* Not all individuals need supplements, consult your health care provider
** ≥ Greater than or equal to

Source: Tufts University; U.S. Department of Agriculture, Department of health and Human Services.

poultry, fish, dry beans, and egg group, the elderly person should consider variety as well as cost and availability. Main dishes made from beans, grains, and vegetables are low in cost and can provide high-quality protein, add fiber to the diet, and help to minimize intake of saturated fat and cholesterol.

*Fiber enhances water absorption, stimulates intestinal activity, and helps to prevent constipation.*

The nutritional requirements for the elderly include at least eight cups (two quarts) of water daily. The fluid needs of older adults are governed by the amount of physical activity, the medications taken, and renal (kidney) function. The recommended two quarts of fluid per day are in addition to any alcohol, coffee, and tea (which have diuretic effects, so they can contribute to dehydration).

Rounding off the optimal approach to geriatric nutrition are the recommended supplements of calcium, vitamin D, and vitamin $B_{12}$. Calcium and vitamin D (which increases calcium absorption) work together to regulate the bone loss associated with aging. Elderly adults' consumption of calcium declines with age, particularly among those who are lactose intolerant. The elderly also experience decreased gastrointestinal absorption of this important element and of vitamin D. This age-related change puts the elderly at risk for osteoporosis, a metabolic brittle-bone disease that affects more women than men. Vitamin $B_{12}$ is essential for the formation of red blood cells. Deficiency of $B_{12}$ accounts for nearly 10 percent of the anemia found in elderly persons.

# Malnutrition Among Older Adults

Physiological and psychosocial aspects of aging affect the nutritional needs of older adults. Good nutrition plays a critical role in maintaining health and function in elderly individuals. Without an adequate consumption of nutrient-dense calories and fluids, eventually malnutrition occurs.

Older adults in varying stages of malnutrition are found in hospitals, in long-term care facilities, and living independently in the community. Nutritional problems that affect older adults have several major causes:

- Protein-energy deficiency
- Inadequate intake of vitamins and trace minerals
- Obesity
- Depression

As these examples imply, the older person's risk for malnutrition is not due entirely to the physiologic changes of aging. Further study reveals that there are individual and overlapping issues. For example, protein deficits occur because of the psychosocial and physical risks identified in Table 3.2.

Vitamin and mineral deficiencies are common in the elderly, especially those in long-term care facilities. The deficiencies can be traced back to low appetite, side effects from pharmaceuticals, and overall environment. For example, people in these facilities have little exposure to sunlight, which is a source of vitamin D. This deficiency is linked to an increased incidence of osteoporosis, since vitamin D is needed for the body to absorb calcium. Many elderly residents take antidepressants or other drugs that cause dry mouth, altered taste, delayed emptying of the stomach, and constipation—all of which affect vitamin and mineral consumption. Vitamin deficiencies are linked to bruising, impaired wound healing, cognitive disorders, urinary tract infections, and fractures.

## Table 3.2 Risks of Protein Deficit

| Psychosocial Risks | Physical Risks |
| --- | --- |
| Limited income | Poor dental health, caries, missing teeth, etc. |
| Social isolation | Surgery |
| Confusion or depression<br>Affects appetite | Polypharmacy<br>Taking medicines that interact in ways that may inhibit the absorption of protein |
| Dementia<br>Causes a tendency to forget to eat and to wander. Requires consumption of psychotropic drugs which can affect appetite | Inability to self-feed |
| Bereavement<br>Causes grief and lack of appetite | Alcoholism |

While obesity is not as acutely serious as the lack of protein, vitamins, or minerals, it does pose hazards associated with the development of breast cancer, diabetes mellitus, and hypertension. Moreover, obesity can cause a major decline in ability to perform routine daily activities, limits motion on weight-bearing joints, and is associated with the development of pressure ulcers.

## Undernutrition Among Hospitalized Elderly

Margaret, age seventy-eight, is a second-day postoperative patient in an orthopedic unit, recovering from hip replacement surgery. She was admitted from a nursing home, where she has been a resident for two years. At mealtimes, a dietary aide sets up her tray and leaves Margaret to feed herself. An hour later, another aide collects Margaret's tray. No one is quite sure how much Margaret eats (or *if* she eats), and she is too confused to tell anyone.

Like Margaret, nearly 60 percent of elderly patients are admitted to acute care facilities undernourished or develop malnutrition during their hospital stay. Health care workers are often unaware of the likelihood that a patient will develop nutritional deficits when conditions prevent eating—as in the routine of instructing patients not to eat before surgery—and no alternative nutrition is ordered. Even after elderly patients are able to resume eating, they may lose their appetites due to physiologic stress caused by wound healing, fever, infection, and pain. Under these conditions, hospital staff can remedy malnutrition by reviewing the patient's nutritional status and daily caloric intake, developing an appropriate high-calorie diet with supplemental feedings, and closely monitoring the patient. Persistent nutritional deficits may indicate a need for more aggressive feeding therapies.

## Undernutrition in Long-Term Care

Nursing home placement is not a guarantee against nutritional risks, because malnutrition in nursing homes is frequently overlooked by physicians, nurses, and caregivers. Between 35 and 50 percent of elderly residents of long-term care facilities are malnourished. The following nutrition-related problems are most common in nursing homes:

- Unintended weight loss
- Dehydration
- Pressure ulcers
- Complications from tube feedings

The causes of malnutrition in nursing homes are complex, and they stem from several diseases and disabilities, including dementia, depression, poor kidney function, cancer, emphysema, heart disease, and impaired ability to self-feed. As with the hospitalized elderly, the aged in long-term care often are admitted to the facility in a poor nutritional state. Residents in these settings typically are taking multiple drugs prescribed for their diseases, and many experience side effects that affect appetite, chewing, swallowing, and other functions of digestion. At mealtimes these frail elders depend on staff supervision to ensure that they have their dentures in, their food cut up, and whatever other assistance they require.

Staff who are caring for residents of long-term care facilities should respect the food preferences of patients who are rapidly losing weight. Other efforts at providing adequate nutrition include offering fortified supplements between meals, encouraging dehydrated patients to drink fluids during the day, regularly repositioning patients with pressure ulcers, and maintaining head elevation in tube-fed patients. Facilities should also weigh all residents weekly to monitor weight loss and gain.

## Undernutrition Among Independent Elders

Ken, eighty-two, was recently widowed. He has limited cooking skills, and supermarkets were just places he drove to when he took his wife shopping. Now he depends on a local convenience store for his marketing, and he tends to buy whatever is easy to carry, since he no longer drives. His diet consists of bread, cereals, pastries, and some easy-to-manage fruit. He supplements this menu with frequent trips to a nearby fast-food restaurant.

Most likely, Ken is among the hundreds of thousands of older adults living independently who are malnourished. By some estimates, the number of homebound elders who are undernourished is as high as a million or more. Older adults in the community display signs of inadequate food intake and the resulting malnutrition for the following reasons:

- Decrease in the senses of taste and smell, often associated with smoking and poor dental health
- Increase in early satiety, or feeling full
- Increased use of both prescription and nonprescription drugs, which may affect appetite and digestion
- Chronic infections and disorders
- Logistical problems in shopping for food, preparing it, and even eating

## Malnutrition and Immune Function

Compared to the population as a whole, the elderly experience greater morbidity and mortality from infections. This apparent susceptibility to infections has been related to the weakening of immune function due to age. Malnutrition contributes to the elderly population's weakened defenses against infections.

Many health problems signal improper nutrition and resulting impairment of the immune system. When older adults are poorly nourished, they are more likely to develop pressure ulcers, experience poor wound healing, and succumb to infections. These conditions occur in elders who are either undernourished or obese.

Failure to consume enough protein and amino acids affects immune status. In people with protein deficiency, the immune function of cells is impaired, and antibody action decreases. Vitamins and minerals also play a fundamental role in immunity in the elderly. For example, the deficiency of vitamin A affects the integrity of mucus-producing cells and retards antibody production. A deficit of vitamin D occurs in elderly persons who have minimal exposure to sunlight and insufficient intake of fortified dairy products. This vitamin acts with calcium to diminish the bone loss associated with aging. Vitamin $B_{12}$ is necessary for the production of red blood cells, and it supports the immune response that acts as a barrier to infections caused by a type of bacteria called *Streptococcus pneumoniae*.

Since aging has long been associated with susceptibility to infections and since we know that sound nutrition helps the body maintain its defense mechanisms, eating well is an obvious way to protect the health of the elderly. To achieve and maintain optimum nutrition, older adults need to adjust their dietary habits to accommodate the different requirements of the aging body.

# Cultural Influences on Nutrition

Lifelong eating habits grow out of cultural traditions, religious influence, and social practices. Food preferences take on emotional overtones as they develop within this context. However, cultural eating habits are not always compatible with optimal nutrition. Health care providers need to understand the relationship between cultural practices and lifestyle in order to modify health care accordingly.

## African-American Elders

The average life expectancy of African-American men and women is less than that of similarly aged whites. The increased mortality among this population is due to excess illness and injury before age sixty-five. African-Americans experience excess mortality from cardiovascular disease, and this finding is one of several attributed to health problems influenced by diet, education, and socioeconomic status.

Nutritional deficiencies resulting in health-related disorders affect many African-Americans. For example, African-American diets typically are low in fruits, vegetables, and whole-grain products. Sodium intake is high, and there are deficiencies in iron and calcium. Lactose intolerance, more common among African-Americans than other Americans, may be partially responsible for lower intake of dairy products. Food preparation practices, notably frying, may also contribute to obesity, another widespread health problem. Diabetes affects almost 20 percent of the African-American population. This fact, combined with the disabilities related to hypertension and stroke, are strong motivations to improve dietary habits.

As an example, foods listed in the Food Guide Pyramid can easily include many African-American (and Southern) favorites. The bread and cereal group includes grits, corn bread, and hominy; the vegetable group would include greens, turnips, sweet potatoes, okra, and coleslaw. These are some ways traditional foods can be used to encourage a healthy nutritional intake.

## Hispanic Elders

The thirty million Hispanic Americans are the second-largest minority group and fastest-growing segment of the U.S. population. They are also the second-poorest minority group and have an overall impaired health status reflecting their low-income status.

Hispanic Americans have less access to health care than other ethnic minorities because most do not have any type of health insurance. When screening services are available for the detection and prevention of disease, Hispanic Americans tend not to use them. One reason offered for this behavior is a language barrier. Hispanics in the United States are at much greater risk for health problems than the general population.

One source of the increased risk is diet. Hispanics generally have a low intake of milk and do not compensate with an increased intake of calcium-rich foods. Hispanic Americans tend to consume cereals infrequently, so their intake of folate and vitamin $B_6$ is below the levels needed to lower risks for vascular disease.

Deficits in folate and vitamin $B_6$ predispose the body to vascular disease. Good food sources of folate include whole grains, dried beans, and green vegetables.

Obesity is a significant problem in Hispanic communities. While the typical Hispanic diet is varied, this group eats processed foods more commonly than fresh foods. Meals tend to be large and calorie laden, and Hispanic consumers are heavy users of fast foods, which are fried and high in sodium and saturated fats. Diabetes is almost three times more common in Puerto Rican and Mexican-American adults than in non-Hispanic whites. It is especially prevalent in the older adult population. About 90 percent of the Hispanics who are diabetic have type II diabetes, which is adult-onset diabetes, caused by impaired insulin secretion and by the body's resistance to the action of insulin. This group suffers high rates of diabetic complications, such as renal (kidney) impairment, retinopathy (an eye disorder), and peripheral vascular disease (diminished circulation in arms and legs).

In light of these risk factors, those who help elderly persons develop diet plans should first assess current dietary practices. A healthful diet should be compatible with cultural food choices.

## Asian-American and Pacific Islander Elders

With little data available on health behaviors of Asian-Americans and Pacific Islander Americans, it is difficult to determine how effectively current health programs are reaching this population. Americans with ancestry from Asia and the Pacific Islands make up about 1.5 percent of the U.S. older-adult population. They trace their origins to more than thirty countries, and as with other immigrant groups, their adaptation to American life affects their health and nutrition.

The mortality rates of this ethnic minority group are lower than among white Americans of similar age. Diet and lifestyle may be responsible for this difference. The first- and second-generation families develop risks for heart disease and some cancers comparable to those of U.S.–born cohorts. Presumably, generations raised in the United States acquire diet and lifestyle patterns that account for this trend.

## Native American Elders

The term *Native American* includes American Indians, Eskimos, and Aleuts. About 6 percent of the Native American population is over the age of sixty-five. According to the Indian Health Service, the average life expectancy for this ethnic minority group is sixty-seven years— eight years less than that of white Americans.

The health and disability problems afflicting Native American elders stem from alcoholism, obesity, diabetes, and hypertension, although alcoholism generally takes its toll before old age. The traditional Native American diet is lower in fat and higher in fiber than typical American meals. However, Native Americans have tended to adopt the more convenient diets, which have contributed to widespread obesity, hypertension, atherosclerosis, and diabetes, along with the complications and disabilities associated with those diseases.

The existence of diabetes is so pervasive—up to 50 percent of the Native American population in some tribes—that an initiative has been proposed and led by the Public Health Service to make prevention and control a tribal responsibility. Tribal leaders, national organizations, and community members are engaged in efforts to educate Native Americans about the seriousness of diabetes and the importance of control. The program also targets youth with messages of healthful eating and exercise.

While there has been improvement in the nutritional status of minorities, the benefits of dietary modifications should be extended to all older adults in ethnic minority groups. However, dietary interventions will succeed only when health care providers respectfully consider cultural and ethnic differences. Social norms and religious practices underlie the traditions and beliefs of minority populations. Ethnic patterns in food preferences are a distinctive means of reinforcing cohesiveness of the group.

# Nutrition Assistance for Elders in the Community

As the population in the United States ages, more programs have been designed to deliver health and related services to the elderly. Several government programs offer assistance to older adults who have limited income and need food, nutritional guidance, or both. These programs include the Elderly Nutrition Program, food stamps, and the Commodity Supplemental Food program.

The Elderly Nutrition Program (ENP) is the largest U.S. community program for older adults. This program is authorized under the

Older Americans Act and administered by the Administration on Aging (AOA). The AOA gives state units on aging Title III-C grants that help them to provide daily meals and related nutrition services in congregate (group) or home settings to people age sixty and older. Title VI established a program for tribal organizations to deliver social and nutritional services to Native Americans, Alaskan Natives, and Native Hawaiians. Participants in these programs receive nutrient-dense meals that provide between 40 and 50 percent of Recommended Dietary Allowances.

The congregate and the home-delivered participants benefit not only from the nutrition, but also from increased social opportunities. The home-delivery contacts are shorter than the social interaction enjoyed by elders at local senior centers or church halls, where many of the meal sites are located. Nevertheless, the majority of the home-delivered participants report that the contact with the delivery person is very important to them socially.

ENP services are targeted to elders in economic or social need, with special attention given to low-income minorities, but there is no income requirement for participation. In addition to providing nutrition and nutrition-related services, the ENP supplies useful links to other community-based services such as homemaker/home health aide services, transportation, fitness programs, and home repair and home modification programs.

The primary source of nutrition assistance for low-income elderly is the *food stamp* program. Food stamps are coupons that consumers redeem for food in stores. Although food stamps can increase the purchasing power of older adults who need this income assistance, many eligible elderly do not participate for several reasons:

- They may not know that the program exists.
- They may feel being "on welfare" has a social stigma.
- They may be misinformed about the program. Many older people assume they are ineligible if they are homeowners or do not have dependent children.
- They may perceive that the application process is too complicated or not worth the effort for what appear to be low benefits.

These barriers to assistance indicate a need for more outreach. Group presentations are an important way to educate the elderly about the food stamp program and thus relieve their doubts. Newspaper features, TV and radio public service announcements, flyers, and brochures also can help publicize programs. The cooperation of other social agencies, such as area agencies on aging and fuel assistance programs, can also facilitate the application process.

The Commodity Supplemental Food program provides supplemental foods to low-income elderly persons. Local sponsors distribute food packages that are labeled to indicate the specific nutritional needs of the elderly. The foods included are canned fruits and vegetables, meats and fish, peanut butter, cereal and grain products, and dairy products.

The website www.benefitscheckup.org is a useful way to determine benefit eligibility. Anyone using this site can screen for public programs and services, and the results are quick and confidential.

# Causes and Consequences of Malnutrition

Ideally, nutrition screening should be incorporated into the clinical care of elderly persons. Nutrition screening ranges from measuring height and weight to examining skin tone, observing behavior, and asking questions about diet. Blood tests and sophisticated assessment techniques are also part of nutrition screening in selected situations. Professional and nonprofessional caregivers can cultivate an increased awareness of the many risk factors that affect the nutritional status of older adults. Caregivers should be particularly watchful for signs of protein-energy malnutrition (also known as protein-calorie malnutrition), which is a deficiency in both macronutrients and micronutrients.

Consider the example of Betty, age eighty-four, who had hip replacement surgery that left her too unsteady to walk unassisted. She lives at home with an unmarried son, who is a schoolteacher. Although Betty spends most of her day in a wheelchair, she maneuvers quite well around her small home. She goes from the bathroom, where she can toilet herself, back to the kitchen, where she empties the dishwasher or folds some laundry that her son leaves in a basket. She keeps a portable phone with her at all times. Her son is relieved that Betty uses the wheelchair, because he feels it provides her with security and stability.

Secretly, he is surprised she remembers to use it, since lately her judgment has been poor. He came home one day to find a burner lit on the stove and the refrigerator door open. Apparently Betty was going to cook something but then forgot all about it. She often forgets to eat but satisfies herself by snacking on a cookie from one of several open boxes left on the kitchen counter. There is still half a layer cake sitting on her kitchen table from last night's supper. In the living room, there are bowls of chocolates that she insists on having "in case someone drops in." She herself doesn't eat them.

One day Betty phoned her son at work because she noticed a trickle of blood running down the front of her leg. A close look at Betty's legs revealed that they were bruised and discolored. The skin, dry and scaly, showed signs of healed skin tears and the one new tear that was bleeding. When Betty's son took her to the emergency department of the local hospital for treatment, he was shocked to hear the physician who dressed the wound call Betty "malnourished." The son admitted to the physician that Betty's appetite is poor, but after months of nagging her to try something more substantial, he had just given up.

Betty displays several of the classic signs of protein calorie malnutrition, an insufficient intake of calories and protein at the expense of a high-carbohydrate, low-protein diet. Those symptoms are weight loss; dry, scaly skin; and loss of muscle mass.

Protein, a nutritive substance found in both vegetable and animal sources, is essential for growth, the building of new tissue, and the repair of injured or broken-down tissue. In particular, muscle is built from protein. Unlike fat cells for fat, or muscle and liver tissue for glucose, there is no place in the body to store protein. Therefore, as the body uses protein, we need to replenish it by consuming adequate amounts of appropriate foods.

Older adults, often limited by the physiologic changes of aging or the progression of disease, are at risk for consuming inadequate protein. Consequently, protein-energy malnutrition is found in older adults living in the community, as well as elders who are residents in long-term care.

Some of the chronic diseases commonly associated with malnutrition in older adults are heart disease, cancer, gastrointestinal disorders, chronic obstructive pulmonary disease, and dementia. The relationship between malnutrition and these diseases is extremely complex. When energy and nutrient needs increase—such as when fever and infection change the body's metabolism—those increased demands on the body can intensify malnutrition. Other conditions that contribute to malnutrition include loss of appetite, difficulty chewing and swallowing, multiple medications, and poor absorption of nutrients.

As part of the medical treatment for malnutrition, the doctor usually places the older-adult patient on a prescribed diet. The dietary instructions typically include a list of foods to avoid. However, unless the instructions are tailored to the individual and the patient is closely monitored, the patient may substitute inappropriate foods, and there will be no nutritional gain. Sometimes the malnutrition is serious enough to require aggressive nutritional intervention. If the elderly patient does not have a terminal illness and if the treatment is likely to improve the quality of life, many physicians feel that the most effective method of nutritional intervention is enteral feeding (tube feeding).

## Weight Loss in Older Adults

Many factors may cause or contribute to unintentional weight loss. The following are among the most commonly observed in elderly persons:

- Acute and chronic illnesses such as gastrointestinal disorders, heart disease, diabetes, and infections
- Psychiatric disorders such as depression and dementia
- Oral and dental problems
- Medications, including withdrawal from some drugs (for example, alcohol or other psychoactives)
- Socioeconomic issues, such as widowhood, poverty, and cultural practices

Table 3.3 lists some medications that can bring about weight loss.

Weight loss is a sensitive and important signal of malnutrition. In many cases unintentional weight loss and low body weight are predictive of the rate of disease and death of older adults. During the normal course of aging, metabolism declines, organ function diminishes,

### Table 3.3 Medications That Can Bring About Weight Loss

| Medications That May Cause Anorexia | Medications That May Cause Nausea | Medications That May Increase Metabolism | Medications That May Cause Malabsorption of Nutrients |
|---|---|---|---|
| Digoxin (prescribed for congestive heart failure or other cardiac conditions) | Antibiotics | Thyroxine or Synthroid (a thyroid hormone) | Sorbitol (vehicle in theophylline elixir) |
| Quinidine or Cardioquin (prescribed for abnormal heart rhythms) | Theophylline or Slophyllin (a bronchodilator) | Theophylline | Cholestyramine or Questran (a blood-fat reducer) |
| Hydralazine or Apresoline (a high blood pressure medication) | Aspirin | | |
| Vitamin A | | | |
| Fluoxetine or Prozac (an antidepressant) | | | |

and muscle tissue is reduced. Nevertheless, the most frequent reasons for unintentional weight loss are acute and chronic illnesses. With the use of individualized diets and calorie-rich, low-volume meals, it is possible to increase weight maintenance or gain in elders. Systematic monitoring of weight loss of the elderly is critical, even of obese elders, because they too may experience weight loss. Even elders who continue to appear overweight may be malnourished.

## Malnutrition and Skin

There is a strong, important link between skin health and nutritional status. A malnourished older adult is at high risk for pressure ulcers, skin tears, and infections caused by breaks in the skin, partly because of nutritional factors and partly because of skin changes due to normal aging.

The nutritional factors that can cause skin breakdown include protein deficiency, anemia, and dehydration. The treatment for the malnourished older adult incorporates a high protein diet with increased caloric content and optimum hydration.

Some of the skin changes caused by normal aging are thinning, a loss of subcutaneous fat, and diminished blood supply. Skin dryness is a common complaint of the elderly, which can be due to nutritional deficiencies, dehydration, or exposure to environmental stresses.

Since dry skin itches and tears easily, older adults are often at risk of jeopardizing their body's first defense against infection. There are several simple measures that can help replenish the skin's moisture and can help it retain moisture:

- Using superfatted soaps
- Using moisturizing ointments or lotions
- Limiting the number of baths or showers taken each week
- Using warm, not hot, water
- Drinking more water throughout the day

## Loss of Muscle Mass

Muscle mass, tone, and strength all diminish as aging progresses. As an adult grows older, his or her body undergoes a slow, progressive loss of nearly 40 percent of muscle tissue. Muscle fibers deteriorate, and collagen replaces the muscle, creating a barrier to oxygen and nutrient supplies.

Loss of muscle tissue affects essential requirements for health and independence: endurance, strength, balance, and flexibility. However, the older adult can maintain or partially restore these four abilities through exercise. Muscle-strengthening techniques involve the basic principles of resistance and progression. This progressive resistive exercise may include weights, mechanical resistance, or just gravity. When an exercise becomes easy, it is time to increase resistance.

Before beginning a fitness program, older adults should seek medical advice. Fortunately, there are exercises available for all who want to increase strength or maintain their fitness level, from the frail, impaired nursing home resident with limited mobility to the vigorous, independent older adult.

## *Gastrointestinal Disorders*

Some gastrointestinal disorders that afflict older adults do not impair normal functioning and may not seem to be serious. Nevertheless, they are very real problems to those older adults who experience them. An example is gastroesophageal reflux disease (GERD). GERD may be the most common digestive disorder seen in clinical practice. The gastric contents regurgitate (or back up) into the esophagus causing the most common symptom, heartburn. Prolonged exposure to stomach acid and digestive enzymes is irritating to the membrane lining the esophagus, which can eventually cause serious damage. It is also associated with increased use of over-the-counter antacid therapy, as many older adults use this method of self-treatment.

Some less common symptoms of GERD include noncardiac chest pain, chronic cough, recurrent pneumonia, nausea, and the erosion of dental enamel. About 50 percent of patients with unexplained chest pain and normal coronary arteries are experiencing heartburn. The reflux of stomach acid in GERD is caused by a relaxing of the lower esophageal sphincter (control valve) and hiatal hernia. The presence of hiatal hernia is not a definite sign of GERD but it is a contributing factor.

## Drugs Associated with Injury to the Esophagus

- Alendronate or Fosamax
- NSAIDs (Advil)
- Potassium replacements, such as Slow-K and KayCiel
- Ferrous sulfate or Feosol
- Tetracycline antibiotics, such as Declomycin

Treatment of GERD begins with lifestyle modifications such as the following measures:

- Elevating the head of the bed
- Lowering fat intake and increasing protein intake
- Avoiding citrus juices, coffee, tomato products, alcohol, and chocolate
- Stopping smoking
- Avoiding potential problem-causing categories of medications (anticholinergics, sedatives, tranquilizers, prostaglandins, calcium-channel blockers)

In addition, two new endoscopic procedures have recently been approved by the Food and Drug Administration for treatment of selected patients with GERD. Both approaches "tighten" the lower esophageal sphincter (LES). One is a suturing technique, and the other uses radio-frequency energy to create scar tissue that helps to shrink the valve near the LES.

## Alcoholism

The degree of alcoholism among the elderly is unclear. However, considering that the fastest-growing segment of the American population is that of persons sixty-five and older, the management of this disorder among the elderly will challenge health care workers more and more as the population of elderly increases.

Upwards of 15 percent of nursing home residents are alcoholic, as are 30 percent or more of those who live in Veterans Administration facilities. These high-risk groups of older adults are prone to adverse drug-alcohol reactions. Since geriatric clients typically ingest seven or eight prescription drugs daily, there are many opportunities for untoward drug effects. Furthermore, alcohol has a damaging effect on the nutrients consumed, so elderly persons who drink are also candidates for malnutrition. Chronic abuse of alcohol impairs the nutritional status of older adults in many ways:

- By decreasing the body's water content, causing dehydration
- By increasing body fat because of alcohol's calorie content

- By decreasing lean body mass as fat replaces muscle
- By suppressing the immune system
- By damaging the central nervous system, contributing to the development of dementia

Alcoholics who start abusing alcohol after the age of sixty are said to have late-onset alcoholism. This form of alcoholism is thought to be a response to some of the changes and losses that affect older adults. The loss of a spouse generates the problem of loneliness, a variety of chronic disorders may cause increasingly numerous physical discomforts, and many elderly experience a decline in economic status. The elderly person may treat alcohol as a way to numb unpleasant feelings associated with these difficulties.

Evidence suggests that health care professionals miss the diagnosis of alcoholism in more than 20 percent of elderly patients admitted to the hospital. Many of the fractures associated with falls are alcohol-related, as are motor vehicle accidents involving impaired elders. This evidence demonstrates the need to educate health care professionals, as well as older adults and their caregivers, in the prevention, recognition, and treatment of geriatric alcoholism.

## Drug Interactions

The concurrent use of many medications, called *polypharmacy*, frequently contributes to malnutrition among the elderly. The types of medication used by the elderly vary with the setting. Elders living in the community most frequently require prescriptions for painkillers, diuretics, cardiovascular drugs, and sedatives. These independent elders also purchase a wide array of over-the-counter drugs for gastrointestinal complaints, nonsteroidal anti-inflammatory drugs (NSAIDs) for their joint pains, and cold remedies. Residents in long-term care most often use antipsychotics and sedative-hypnotics followed by diuretics, antihypertensives, analgesics, cardiac drugs, and antibiotics. Long-term care residents ingest an average of eight medications daily. Of the drugs used most frequently, twenty-three are known to cause reduced food intake and to have such side effects as anorexia, nausea, vomiting, constipation, drowsiness, and lack of interest in or aversion to food.

Polypharmacy increases the risk of drug-induced malnutrition due to alteration of appetite as well as the absorption and metabolism of nutrients. Psychotropic drugs (and others) frequently affect the physical and mental well-being of an individual, often before blood levels of nutrients show reduced levels. When caregivers have questions about nutrient-drug interactions, they should consult with the physician, pharmacist, and dietitian. To counteract the effects of drugs on nutrition, caregivers should also accommodate the food preferences of elderly persons.

## Oral Health

A century ago, tooth loss by middle age was not only common, but accepted as the norm. Since then, there have been many developments in improving oral health, ranging from community water fluoridation to better methods of detecting dental problems. Even so, there is what has been called a "silent epidemic" of dental and oral disease. The Surgeon General's document "Healthy People 2010" included the following facts about oral health among the nation's elderly:

- Among adults between the ages of sixty-five and seventy-four, 23 percent have severe periodontal disease.
- Oral and pharyngeal (mouth and throat) cancers are found in about 30,000 adults each year. They are primarily diagnosed in the elderly.
- Most elderly take several medications, and nursing home residents take an average of eight prescription drugs daily. A common side effect, dry mouth, increases the chance of oral disease.

The mouth is a reliable indicator of general health. Recent research findings have linked heart and lung diseases, diabetes, and stroke to chronic oral infections. There is a significant association between malnutrition and the oral health of the older adult. More specifically, the following detrimental oral conditions are associated with nutritional deficiency in elderly persons:

- Wearing poorly fitting dentures
- Not wearing dentures when tooth loss exists
- Dental caries
- Periodontal disease
- Dry mouth
- Pain

An older adult with one or more of these problems may eliminate foods that are difficult to chew or swallow. The more foods eliminated from the diet, the greater the likelihood of developing nutritional deficiencies. The deficiencies then affect the mouth, teeth, and gums, thus starting another potentially serious cycle of deteriorating nutritional status.

Tooth loss is considered a general measurement to help evaluate the amount of severe oral health problems in adults. More than half of older adults over eighty have lost all their natural teeth. Among nursing home residents, 30 to 80 percent who have lost their teeth are affected by swallowing impairments. Lack of assessment or effective treatment for these conditions are avoidable causes of malnutrition in nursing home residents.

Normal saliva flow is necessary for oral health because it buffers the acid produced by bacteria and mechanically cleanses the mouth. Most age-related changes in salivary function result from illnesses or their treatment. Nearly one in five older adults experiences dry mouth (xerostomia), which is a common side effect of some diseases and medications.

*Problems caused by dry mouth include periodontal disease, difficulty in chewing and swallowing, unpleasant taste sensation, and impaired food enjoyment.*

Poor oral health is an important and potentially reversible contributing factor to significant involuntary weight loss. However, it is difficult to find substantial correlations among tooth loss, nutritional status, and compromised health. Whether this is because our modern diet is primarily made up of soft, processed foods that do not require much chewing or because data and collection methods are inadequate is unclear. However, we do know that malnutrition can and does contribute to physical and mental decline. A recent investigation of U.S. nursing homes declared malnutrition, dehydration, and weight loss in long-term care to be an insidious and widespread problem. Inadequate staffing is cited as the primary contributing factor.

# Nutritional Choices

Some of the barriers to meeting the nutritional needs of older adults living independently are economic limitations, transportation problems, inability to carry groceries, depression, and dementia. Yet, to some degree, elders can control their nutritional intake, and in doing so, they can maximize their level of wellness. Awareness requires learning what foods are nutrient-dense and what foods simply provide empty calories and contain high amounts of fats, sugar, and salt. As older adults expand their knowledge of food, they can set realistic nutritional goals and improve overall health and well-being. Elderly nursing home residents who are able to make food selections should be encouraged and helped to do so.

Food service is a key component of the long-term care setting. A good food program not only meets a fundamental human need, but it also is an extremely important element in any resident's overall quality of life.

# 4

# Pharmacology and the Older Adult

THE INCREASING LONGEVITY of Americans and the aging of the baby boomer generation are constant reminders that the American population is becoming older. Some of the increased attention paid to medical issues, health policies, and social concern has been devoted to the appropriate use of medication by the elderly. Aging is often related to more frequent chronic illness (often combined with multiple health problems) and an increased use of medications. Becoming older does not necessarily lead to increasing illness, but aging is associated with anatomical and physiological changes that affect how the body metabolizes medications. Therefore, maintaining and improving the health of older people requires an understanding of the absorption, distribution, metabolism, and excretion of drugs and of the body's responses to these medications.

## Drug Use by Older Adults

Elderly Americans frequently use several drugs concurrently. Ninety percent of Americans over the age of sixty-five take at least one prescription medication daily, and most take two or more. In long-term care facilities, two-thirds of the residents receive three or more drugs daily, with an average of seven or eight different medications per patient. These older adults are at increased risk for adverse drug reactions because of their multiple diseases, altered ability to metabolize and excrete the products of their complex medication regimen, and possible sensory and cognitive deficits. Some of the predominant reactions are lethargy, confusion, gastrointestinal disturbances, and falls.

The commonly used drugs among the elderly living in the community are cardiovascular drugs, antihypertensive agents, analgesics, anti-inflammatory drugs, sedatives, and gastrointestinal preparations.

Polypharmacy—taking several medications concurrently—increases the potential for adverse drug reactions, that is, any unintended, undesirable response to a medication. The chances of an elderly person experiencing an adverse drug reaction are two to three times higher than in a younger adult. Unfortunately, this is probably an underestimate, because many caregivers—and indeed most older adults living independently—fail to recognize adverse reactions, attributing such symptoms to characteristics of "old age." In addition, there is a scarcity of data available in this specialized area. Few researchers have formally explored the relationship between under prescribing and health-related outcomes in institutionalized patients.

Many of the problems generated by polypharmacy are triggered by elderly patients seeking care by visiting a different physician for each of their problems. This approach makes it more difficult to consider *pharmacodynamics* (what drugs do to the body) and *pharmacokinetics* (what the body does to the ingested drugs). These two processes are associated with the following changes:

- Extended duration of medication activity
- Increased or decreased drug effect
- Potential for drug toxicity
- Increased opportunity for adverse drug reaction

Reducing the incidence of polypharmacy is a health protection goal of "Healthy People 2010," a statement of national health objectives published by the U.S. Department of Health and Human Services. Older adults, particularly older women living independently, are at highest risk for complications of polypharmacy. These complications result from the combination of age-related changes in pharmacokinetics and pharmacodynamics, the presence of multiple illnesses requiring treatment with medications, and high rates of noncompliance (unintentional or not) with their therapeutic regimen. (Noncompliance is a patient's deviation from the treatment plan, as when a patient fails to take medicine or takes the wrong dose.)

# *Pharmacokinetics: What Metabolism Does to the Drugs*

The process of aging changes the way the body metabolizes medications. Pharmacokinetics is influenced by the aging process in several ways, summarized in Table 4.1. In general, the body may become less effective in absorbing, metabolizing, and eliminating drugs. The increase in body fat and decrease in volume of water in the body alters drug distribution patterns. This change affects the length of time the drug is active in the body.

### Table 4.1 How Aging Changes the Way the Body Processes Drugs

| Process | Change | Example |
|---|---|---|
| Absorption | Mucosal surface decreases; intestinal blood flow declines; secretion of gastric (stomach) acid decreases | Absorption of calcium, iron, and thiamine is reduced. |
| Distribution | Lean body mass decreases; adipose (fatty) tissue increases; fat-soluble drugs prolonged | Sedatives, such as barbiturates and some benzodiazepines remain in the body longer. Digoxin, a cardiac drug used to strengthen the heart, also remains in the body longer, which can cause toxicity. |
| Metabolism | Liver decreases in size; blood flow to liver declines. | The ability of the liver to break down such drugs as calcium-channel blockers, tricyclic antidepressants, warfarin, and phenytoin is affected and they may not be eliminated as easily. |
| Elimination | Renal (kidney) function declines; renal size and blood flow decrease. | Can significantly affect therapeutic response of digoxin, lithium, and aminoglycosides. |

## *Pharmacodynamics: How Drugs Affect the Body*

In contrast to pharmacokinetics (how the body processes drugs), scientists know much less about pharmacodynamics (the way drugs affect the body) in elderly patients. However, we do have information about changes detected in the action of several drugs. For example, research has demonstrated that there is an increased receptor response for several commonly used medications:

- *Benzodiazepines*—These sedatives cause greater drowsiness in elderly patients.
- *Opiates*—In elderly patients, opiates provide stronger pain control and are more likely to cause problems with breathing.
- *Warfarin*—This anticoagulant produces a stronger response in elderly patients, causing bleeding complications.

Reviewing the physical changes in older adults and the effects of these changes on the metabolism of drugs clearly demonstrates the likelihood for adverse drug reactions. Furthermore, as a group, the elderly are more likely to endure multiple chronic illnesses that require several medications. As the number of prescriptions increases, so does the potential for problems caused by drug interactions.

## Drugs Predominantly Used in Long-Term Care

- Laxatives
- Analgesics
- Sedatives/hypnotics
- Neuroleptics (drugs for modifying psychotic behavior)

Not only does the geriatric population have a large number of illnesses, creating a higher level of drug consumption and side effects, but many of the side effects resemble illnesses. Doctors observing these side effects may diagnose illnesses and prescribe still more drugs. The table lists the drugs that are most commonly prescribed for older adults and the potential for adverse reactions. Older adults need to give their doctors accurate histories of drug consumption, so their doctors can recognize side effects for what they are. Otherwise, they risk consuming yet another drug with another potential side effect.

## Potential Hazards

Generally, polypharmacy is associated with a high incidence of adverse drug reactions and drug interactions among the elderly. The physical changes of aging, multiple illnesses, and multiple prescriptions to treat these illnesses place older adults in a high-risk category.

Adverse drug responses among older adults who live in the community are difficult to document with any precision, because the patient may not recognize an unusual physical or mood occurrence or may attribute it to aging. As a result, the event will probably be minimized or may even go unreported. Adverse drug reactions in the elderly may not manifest themselves in the "typical" manner, causing clinicians to ascribe physical or emotional complaints solely to aging, rather than to an unwanted drug effect.

## Medication Errors

There are many causes of medication errors. One of the most common of these is the overall lack of knowledge about drug therapy. This inevitably leads to inappropriate prescribing, inappropriate drug delivery, inappropriate patient behavior, and inappropriate drug monitoring.

Contributing to this problem, many drug clinical trials are biased. The trials frequently exclude the elderly population because investigators believe that older adults, more often than younger adults, may experience toxicity with the test drug. For example, patients over the age of seventy-five have often been routinely omitted from clinical trials of drugs for high blood pressure and anti-clotting drugs for heart attack patients.

### Table 4.2 Drugs and Their Potential for Adverse Reactions

| Classification | Drug | Caution |
|---|---|---|
| Cardiovascular | Digoxin | Usual symptoms of toxicity are nausea, anorexia, and visual disturbance. May also cause irregular heartbeat. When combined with diuretics, can cause kidney damage if the kidneys are already functioning at diminished capacity. |
| Antihypertensives | Thiazides | Increased potassium loss. Ineffective where there is moderate kidney dysfunction. |
| | Beta-blockers | Although effective and well tolerated in most elderly, can cause problems in patients with peripheral arterial disease by increasing claudication (severe calf pain caused by inadequate blood supply to lower extremities) and in diabetics by extending the duration of hypoglycemia. |
| Anti-inflammatory drugs | NSAIDs | Individual variation in effectiveness; antiplatelet effect, which prevents platelets from performing clotting functions; also may cause gastrointestinal problems. |
| Sedatives | Benzodiazepines | Drugs accumulate in the body; lethargy and confusion likely; falls occur. |
| Neuroleptics, reduce agitated behavior | Phenothiazines, thioxanthenes, and butyrophenones | May cause increased confusion, urinary retention, abnormally low blood pressure, and tardive dyskinesia (involuntary facial tics, tongue and jaw movements, chewing, and rocking or marching). |
| Gastrointestinal aids | Histamine antagonists | May affect the central nervous system: confusion, delirium, slurred speech, etc. |

There is strong evidence that technology could help prevent many prescribing errors. For example, many physicians have begun using computerized prescribing with a personal digital assistant (PDA) or handheld computer. Two immediate advantages of such a tool are that the pharmacist will not misread the physician's handwriting and the technology gives the physician access to immediate feedback about drug information and dosages while writing the prescription.

Pharmacists suggest that physicians indicate medication *use* on their prescriptions. This information adds the benefit of checks and balances. If the pharmacist had any doubt about the name of the drug, the information about its intended use would provide clarification.

Patients also play a role in preventing medication errors. Nearly 20 percent of preventable errors are caused by clinicians not having enough information about the patient, such as age, weight, allergies, and diagnosis. Patients should volunteer this information if the doctor does not ask. Also, patients need to know how to protect themselves from errors by learning correct dosages, drug-food and drug-drug interactions, and possible side effects.

Following prescription of any drug, careful monitoring is important in order to assess the effects of medications and the course of the patient's disease. Basic methods of monitoring include reading vital signs and interpreting laboratory values as they relate to the illness.

Nearly one-third of all preventable adverse effects are related to communication problems, that is, how drug information is distributed. Other sources of errors relate to staff competency, improper storage of drugs, and lack of standard times for administering drugs.

# Medication Problems in Long-Term Care

Long-term care requires different skills than does acute care. Elderly residents are among the frailest of the population, and these ill elders may need to use more medication. Therefore, increased use of medication in this population is appropriate.

Some of the drugs used are thought to offer benefits that outweigh potential risks. For example, although the elderly have an increased sensitivity to benzodiazepines, a group of drugs used as antianxiety and sleep-inducing agents, lorazepam (Ativan) is useful for reducing the anxiety present in many patients with dementia.

Other drugs are thought to offer inadequate benefits or to pose so much risk to the older resident in the nursing home that they are rarely suitable. An example is another benzodiazepine, flurazepam (Dalmane), which takes an extremely long time to break down in the body. It leads to increased sedation and weakness, placing patients at risk for falls.

Data on appropriate drug use in the elderly population are scarce, and more investigation in this area is needed. Nevertheless, the suitable use of medications in nursing home residents is an issue of increasing importance in the care of the elderly, and reducing inappropriate use may be one of the best and most cost-effective ways to improve the quality of care in nursing homes. Several measures are possible:

- *Nondrug alternatives*—The frail elderly residents in long-term care have many disorders for which multiple medications are prescribed, so they are always exposed to hazardous interactions and side effects. In some cases, however, nondrug alternatives are practical. For example dietary modification is usually as effective as laxatives for correcting constipation. Often, the only changes needed are to add bran for fiber intake and to increase fluid consumption. Prompt attention to the toileting needs of the resident also helps to establish a regular elimination schedule.
- *Establishing the correct diagnosis*—Depression is common in the nursing home setting, yet other conditions, including hypothyroidism, mimic the symptoms of depression. Obviously, an antidepressant is not an appropriate prescription for someone whose problem is hypothyroidism. Thorough evaluation of the resident is critical in order to establish a correct diagnosis. Part of this evaluation is a comprehensive drug history.
- *Defining the therapeutic goal*—Treatment should also include a goal for the medication, so that there is a standard for determining whether the patient should discontinue a medication. For example, if an infection is not responding to the prescribed antibiotic in a given period of time, the ineffective medication should be discontinued and a new treatment plan developed.

- *Initial drug therapy*—The initial drug therapy should be at low doses, with gradual increases as needed.

The cause of a disease and degree of disability are both physical and social, and these factors profoundly affect the individual patient's response to drug therapy. Care of residents in nursing homes includes maintenance and increase of function, and to the extent they are reasonable, preventing disease and reducing risks. All these factors directly influence the elderly person's quality of life and functional capacity.

# Inappropriate Medication Use in the Community

Drugs whose adverse risks outweigh their health benefits are inappropriate, yet recent investigations uncovered data showing that the prevalence of inappropriate drug use in the elderly might be higher than expected. But although we have evidence that 40 percent of nursing home patients receive one or more inappropriate drugs, data on inappropriate medication use in community-dwelling older adults are scarce. Earlier studies focused only on groups whose medical records could be systematically monitored—for example, institutionalized elders, hospitalized patients, and clinic outpatients.

The frequency of inappropriate drug use in community-dwelling elders is thought to be slightly lower than that of nursing home residents. The most important factor predicting the likelihood of inappropriate medication use is the total number of prescription medications. The most important subjective characteristic related to unsuitable drug use is the presence of depressive symptoms. This was attributed to the fact that the depressed elderly persons were often misdiagnosed and then prescribed long-acting benzodiazepines. Since depressive symptoms in the elderly are often undetected in an office visit, it is possible that these depressed patients received long-acting benzodiazepines rather than specific antidepressive therapy. If this practice is occurring, not only are community-residing older adults with depressive symptoms receiving the wrong prescription (benzodiazepine), but they are receiving inadequate treatment for depressive disease.

# Noncompliance

In this context, *compliance* refers to the extent to which a patient's behavior keeps pace with the clinician's planned medical regimen. In contrast, as noted earlier, drug noncompliance occurs when there is a deviation from the plan. Noncompliance may be intentional or accidental, and it takes several forms:

- Omitting drugs
- Taking medicines for the wrong reason
- Increasing or decreasing dosages from the prescribed levels
- Using drugs prescribed for someone else

In a study of chronically ill patients in an ambulatory veterans' clinic, only 20 percent were in full compliance with their medication regimen. According to the records of another group of elderly patients, 44 percent were found to be taking prescription medications without the knowledge of their physicians.

## *Reasons for Noncompliance*

Other investigators have shown that among the elderly, 70 percent of noncompliance resulted from patients' *intentional* decisions on how to take medications. Such decisions were based on a fear of side effects and a lack of understanding of both the disease and the importance of the drug prescribed. Because recovery from a chronic illness often reaches a leveling-off point, some patients will try unauthorized medicines and treatments suggested by friends or relatives, simply because it worked for someone *they* knew. It appears that patients make decisions for themselves based on their *perception* of what works. Rather than being willful or seeking attention, the evidence is that noncompliant patients probably have a misperception of their disease and their prescribed medications. They act upon this faulty information in ways that seem to them to be rational.

For example, Albert, eighty-one, lives alone. A year ago, he suffered a stroke but was left with only minor residual effects. He seemed to be successfully maintaining his independence with interim help from his family. Albert's chief complaints were episodes of unsteadiness when he walked and impaired hand grasps.

One day a friend remarked that he could purchase a codeine and aspirin preparation, an analgesic, from another country without a prescription. This sounded like a good idea to Albert, so he gave the neighbor some money and said, "Get some for me."

When questioned by his worried daughter, Albert said he did not know why his neighbor needed the drug. More to the point, Albert also denied having any pain—which is the main reason for taking an analgesic. In spite of this apparent confusion about the drug, he did not understand his daughter's concern and still insisted that it "might help" him.

There are many other reasons for noncompliance. The primary factor is poor communication, which contributes to errors. A patient may be unclear as to how to take the drug. To minimize such risk, patients and their primary caregivers must ask for specific instructions, including precautions. The clinician's responsibility includes providing clear and understandable directions when communicating with patients. In a recent survey of older adults, however, only 12 percent of respondents said they used information sheets from pharmacists, and only 14 percent used instructions from a doctor or nurse to help them increase medicine compliance.

Patients with cognitive, functional, or sensory impairments are often noncompliant. Several tools are available to help older adults with a degree of memory loss to take their medications correctly. These include plastic, compartmentalized pillboxes, blister packs, and containers that beep and can be preset by the pharmacist to indicate when it is time to take a dose. Beepers and wrist alarms do the same. However, these helpful devices almost always need to be used in association with a caregiver.

Functional impairments that contribute to noncompliance range from vision and hearing impairments to arthritis, which limits older adults' ability to manipulate syringes, bottles of eye drops, and safety caps on pill containers. Those with poor vision will need instructions written in large, bold print. The hearing impaired obviously will have difficulty following spoken instructions. Therefore, before giving oral instructions, the clinician will need an initial assessment of the individual's hearing ability in order to learn how severe the deficit is.

Another reason for noncompliance is inappropriate route of administration (prescribing medicine that is difficult for a patient to take—for example, too hard to swallow). If a pill cannot be crushed, the patient who has difficulty swallowing tablets would do better with medication in liquid form. Also, an increasing number of drugs can be ordered as skin patches. This transdermal route of administration is accurate and noninvasive and helps a patient to adhere to a drug regimen.

Patients may fail to comply if they lack knowledge or insight about the need for continued, committed adherence to their pharmaceutical plan. Diabetics and people with mental illness frequently stop taking their medicines once they are feeling better. In these instances, the illness will surely worsen.

A serious barrier for older adults on a fixed income is lack of funds for consistently filling prescriptions. When the choice is food, rent, or a prescription, the patient frequently omits the drug.

## Measures to Improve Compliance

Noncompliance with prescription drug regimens is the predominant health care concern in the United States. Since most patients take their medications incorrectly, it is no wonder that poor compliance is the primary reason for drug failure. Not only is noncompliance lethal in many situations, but it also causes delayed recovery, lost productivity, unnecessary doctor visits, and hospital admissions. All of these grossly inflate health care costs.

The following measures can contribute to patient compliance:

- The doctor and other caregivers should involve the patient in treatment decisions.
- Doctors, physician's assistants, and nurses should monitor compliance each time they see the patient. If needed, they should follow up outside of scheduled visits.

- Health care providers should document patient compliance, using a monitoring form that can be incorporated in the patient's record.
- Caregivers should coordinate patients' medication regimens with other health professionals providing care, such as nurses, physicians' assistants, and pharmacists.
- Development of communication skills should be included in medical training and continuing-education curricula, as well as extended to other health team members to ensure continuity of care.

# Economic Issues of Prescription Therapy

Although drugs continue to be one of the most cost-effective treatment strategies, over 15 percent of geriatric patients who use prescription drugs are unable to pay for them. Prescription drugs are not covered under Medicare. However, some health maintenance organizations and commercial insurance plans do cover part of their costs, and Medicaid covers prescription drugs.

Recent investigation by researchers at Boston University School of Public Health revealed that Americans paid 32 percent more than Canadians for the same drugs in the early 1990s. Surveys by state-based groups show that on average, older adults are being charged double the retail price charged by prescription drug makers to their most favored customers.

Since many elderly adults pay the entire cost of their drugs themselves, this expenditure represents a significant budget item. It is therefore essential to make drug therapy as cost-effective as possible. Clinicians can help in several ways:

- Determine the cost of the geriatric client's medications. For drugs that are within the same therapeutic class and have similar efficacy and toxicity profiles, prescribe the least costly alternative.
- Use generic drugs when possible.

- When assessing whether the patient will be likely to continue using the drug, prescribe a small quantity.
- Assess the suitability of each medication in the drug regimen, and discontinue any unnecessary drugs.
- Use the lowest dose necessary.

In a 1995 landmark study titled *Drug-Related Morbidity and Mortality: A Cost-of-Illness Model*, researchers developed an economic model to estimate the cost of medication-related problems in the ambulatory care population. The researchers took the perspective of a third-party payer looking at various positive and negative outcomes associated with medication therapy. The costs of medication-related illness and death were estimated at $76.6 billion annually. Hospitalizations to treat these drug-related illnesses accounted for the majority of costs, $47 billion. The report shows that monitoring drug therapy is important both medically and economically on a massive scale.

# Alcohol and Drug Abuse

According to a report by the Center for Substance Abuse Treatment/Substance Abuse and Mental Health Services Administration, alcohol abuse and the abuse of legal drugs affect 17 percent of adults age sixty and older. The report goes on to note that a third of those elders who abuse alcohol did not have an alcohol abuse problem when they were younger. The implication is that conditions or situations encountered by the older adult during the aging process are responsible for this destructive behavior.

The elderly may be especially apt to mix drugs and alcohol, and they are at increased risk for the adverse consequences of such combinations. Although persons aged sixty-five and older constitute only 13 percent of the population, they consume more than 30 percent of all prescription medications. Elderly persons are more vulnerable than younger adults to the side effects of drugs, and these events tend to escalate in severity with advancing age. Among persons aged sixty or older, more than 10 percent of those in the community and 40 percent of those in nursing homes fulfill criteria for alcohol abuse.

Several alcohol-drug interactions include:

- An acute dose of alcohol (a single drink or several drinks over several hours) may inhibit a drug's metabolism by competing with the drug for the same set of metabolizing enzymes. This interaction prolongs and enhances the drug's *availability* (the extent to which the administered dose of the drug reaches its site of action), potentially increasing the patient's risk of experiencing harmful side effects from the drug.
- Long-term or chronic alcohol ingestion may activate drug-metabolizing enzymes, resulting in a decrease in the drug's availability and diminishing its effects. After these enzymes have been activated, they remain—even in the absence of alcohol—and continue to affect the metabolism of certain drugs after several weeks of cessation of drinking. Thus, a recently abstinent chronic drinker may need higher doses of medications than those required by nondrinkers to achieve therapeutic levels of certain drugs. In addition, enzymes activated by chronic alcohol consumption transform some drugs into toxic chemicals that can damage the liver or other organs.
- Alcohol can magnify the inhibitory effects of sedative and narcotic drugs at their sites of action in the brain.

Anesthetics are administered prior to surgery to render a patient unconscious and insensitive to pain. Chronic alcohol consumption increases the risk of regurgitation and aspiration (sucking into the lungs) of stomach contents. Other risks are blood coagulation problems, fluid imbalances, and impaired liver function. Alcohol also increases the risk of liver damage that may be caused by certain anesthetics.

Antibiotics are used to treat infectious diseases. In combination with acute alcohol consumption, some antibiotics may cause nausea, vomiting, headache, and possibly convulsions. Among these antibiotics are furazolidone, griseofulvin, metronidazole, and the antimalarial quinacrine. Isoniazid and rifampin are used together to treat tuberculosis, a disease especially problematic among the elderly and among homeless alcoholics. Acute alcohol consumption decreases the availability of isoniazid in the bloodstream, whereas chronic alcohol use decreases the availability of rifampin. In each case, the effectiveness of the medication may be reduced.

Warfarin, an anticoagulant, is commonly prescribed to retard the blood's clotting ability. Acute alcohol consumption enhances warfarin's availability, thereby increasing the patient's risk for life-threatening hemorrhages. Chronic alcohol consumption reduces warfarin's availability, decreasing the patient's protection from the consequences of blood-clotting disorders.

Alcoholism and depression are frequently associated, a fact that leads to high alcohol-antidepressant interactions. Alcohol increases the sedative effect of tricyclic antidepressants such as amitriptyline, impairing mental skills required for driving. Acute alcohol consumption increases the availability of some tricyclics, potentially increasing their sedative effects. Chronic alcohol consumption appears to increase the availability of some tricyclics and to decrease the availability of others. The significance of these interactions is unclear. What is known, however, is that these chronic effects persist in recovering alcoholics. Tyramine, a chemical found in some beers and wine, interacts with some antidepressants such as monoamine oxidase inhibitors, to produce a dangerous rise in blood pressure. As little as one standard drink might cause this interaction.

Oral hypoglycemic drugs are prescribed to help lower blood sugar levels in some patients with diabetes. Acute alcohol consumption decreases the availability of one such drug, tolbutamide. Alcohol also interacts with some drugs of this class to produce symptoms of nausea and headache such as those described for metronidazole.

Antihistamines such as diphenhydramine are available without prescription to treat allergic symptoms and insomnia. Alcohol may intensify the sedation caused by some antihistamines. These drugs can cause excessive dizziness and sedation in older persons. The effects of combining alcohol and antihistamines may therefore be especially significant in this population.

Drugs such as chlorpromazine are used to diminish psychotic symptoms such as delusions and hallucinations. Acute alcohol consumption increases the sedative effect of these drugs, resulting in impaired coordination and potentially fatal breathing difficulties. The combination of chronic alcohol ingestion and antipsychotic drugs may also damage the liver.

Anticonvulsants are prescribed mainly to treat epilepsy. Acute alcohol consumption increases the availability of anticonvulsants, including phenytoin, and the risk of drug-related side effects. Chronic alcoholism may decrease phenytoin availability, significantly reducing the patient's protection against epileptic seizures, even during a period of abstinence.

The commonly prescribed antiulcer medications cimetidine and ranitidine increase the availability of a low dose of alcohol under some circumstances. The clinical significance of this finding is uncertain, since other studies have questioned such interaction at higher doses of alcohol.

Cardiovascular medications include a wide variety of drugs prescribed to treat disorders of the heart and circulatory system. Acute alcohol consumption interacts with some of these drugs to cause vertigo or fainting upon standing up. These drugs include nitroglycerin, used to treat angina, and reserpine, methyldopa, and hydralazine, used to treat hypertension. Chronic alcohol consumption decreases the availability of propranolol (used to treat hypertension), potentially reducing its therapeutic effect.

Narcotic pain relievers are prescribed for moderate to severe pain. They include the opiates morphine, codeine, propoxyphene, and meperidine. The combination of opiates and alcohol intensifies the sedative effect of both substances, increasing the risk of death from overdose. A single dose of alcohol can increase the availability of propoxyphene, potentially increasing its sedative side effects.

Aspirin and aspirin-containing compounds are nonprescription pain relievers commonly used by the elderly. Some of these drugs cause stomach bleeding and inhibit blood from clotting; alcohol can exacerbate these effects. Older persons who mix alcoholic beverages with large doses of aspirin to self-medicate for pain are therefore at particularly high risk for episodes of gastric bleeding. In addition, aspirin may increase the availability of alcohol, heightening the effects of a given dose of alcohol.

Acetaminophen (sold under the brand Tylenol) is a favorite non-aspirin pain reliever used by older adults. Chronic alcohol ingestion activates enzymes that transform acetaminophen into chemicals that can cause liver damage, even when acetaminophen is used in standard therapeutic amounts. These effects may occur with as little as 2.6 grams of acetaminophen in persons consuming widely varying amounts of alcohol.

Benzodiazepines are generally prescribed to treat anxiety and insomnia. Because of their greater safety margin, they have largely replaced barbiturates, which are now used mostly in the emergency treatment of convulsions. Doses of benzodiazepines that are excessively sedating may cause severe drowsiness in the presence of alcohol, increasing the risk of household and automotive accidents. This may be especially true in older people, who demonstrate an increased response to these drugs. Low doses of flurazepam interact with low doses of alcohol to impair driving ability, even when the alcohol is ingested the morning *after* taking flurazepam. Since alcoholics often suffer from anxiety and insomnia, and since many of them take morning drinks, this interaction is dangerous. The benzodiazepine lorazepam is being used increasingly for its antianxiety and sedative effects. Combining alcohol and lorazepam is strongly discouraged.

Acute alcohol consumption increases the availability of barbiturates, prolonging their sedative effect. Chronic alcohol consumption decreases barbiturate availability through enzyme activation. In addition, acute or chronic alcohol consumption enhances the sedative effect of barbiturates at their site of action in the brain, sometimes leading to coma or respiratory failure.

# Underused Drugs

Based on the types of illness present in the U.S. elderly population, we can estimate the kinds of medicine they should be using. Compared to those estimates, evidence suggests that certain kinds of drugs are underused. Some categories of drugs that are particularly underused are medicines for cardiovascular disease, pain medications, and immunizations.

## Medicines That Treat Cardiovascular Disease

There is current evidence that indicates that two statins, simvastatin and pravastatin, reduce overall mortality and have proven long-term safety in those at risk for heart attacks. According to the most recent statistics, statins can reduce cholesterol levels by about sixty points and lessen the chances of heart attacks by about one-third. Statins have been suggested for patients with elevated levels of LDL cholesterol since 1993, and in the succeeding years, the evidence for these drugs has gotten stronger.

However, despite the research and widespread advertising, at least 20 million Americans at risk for heart attacks are not getting these potentially lifesaving drugs. Doctors are prescribing statins for about one in five patients who need them. Surveys conducted between 1990 and 1996 indicated that only 14 percent of those diagnosed with cardiovascular disease received prescriptions for a cholesterol-lowering drug. Currently, between 4.5 and 5 million Americans are taking statins, while at least 25 million more could benefit.

There are several reasons that statins are underprescribed. Many women think heart disease will not harm them (even though heart problems are the number one killer of women). Men often believe they will be given all the treatment they need after they have a heart attack, so they don't ask enough questions about further treatment. Other justifications for the lack of statin use are economic; the drugs are expensive, costing from $75 to $100 per month. In addition, concerns linger about the drugs' safety, despite the latest data suggesting they are safe and produce few side effects. Moreover, doctors are generally conservative and slow to adopt new ideas such as the use of statins. Finally, patients with no outward symptoms of heart trouble are often reluctant to take drugs, like statins, that don't make them feel better.

Thrombolytic therapy is the use of certain drugs called thrombolytics ("clot busters") in heart attack victims within *one hour* of the onset of symptoms. These drugs break up the clot, an action which limits the damage to the heart muscle. The timeliness of the treatment is in direct proportion to the success of the therapy—the longer the delay, the less successful the outcome.

Studies have shown that thrombolytic therapy in elderly patients with multiple health problems is not given as promptly as it is in other heart attack victims. One reason for the delay might be the fact that older adults require more complex assessments because of their many impairments.

Although it can be useful, there are several reasons why this therapy is underutilized in elderly patients. All elderly patients are at high risk for bleeding with this therapy. The older the patient, the greater the chance for hemorrhage with thrombolytic treatment. In addition, thrombolytic therapy cannot be used in recent stroke patients or in patients who have had recent gastrointestinal bleeding. Patients who are receiving anticoagulant therapy or who have had surgery within six or seven days should also avoid this treatment.

Drugs called beta-blockers help to slow the heart rate and to control an irregular heartbeat. Patients sixty-five and older who receive beta-blockers following a heart attack are less likely to die within two years and less likely to be rehospitalized than elderly patients who do not receive this therapy following a heart attack. Despite evidence from several clinical trials, follow-up studies have shown that physicians prescribe these agents to only 30 to 50 percent of patients after a heart attack. According to the records of 200,000 patients who had myocardial infarction, only half of the patients received beta-blockers when they were discharged from the hospital. Those least likely to receive this therapy were patients who were very elderly, black, or considered to be the sickest.

The same studies investigated the reasons for physician reluctance to prescribe beta-blockers. The results suggested that the reluctance is associated with patient characteristics that some physicians presume are contraindications: older age, use of diuretics, history of chronic obstructive pulmonary disease, and poor cardiac function.

Another cardiovascular drug therapy that is underutilized is the use of angiotensin converting enzyme (ACE) inhibitors. Research has confirmed that this therapy benefits patients who have experienced heart failure or a recent heart attack. ACE inhibitors are the only medical therapy to date that has been shown in multiple large trials to alleviate symptoms and prolong life in patients with congestive heart failure. In the past, digoxin, diuretics, and vasodilator therapy formed the primary basis for the treatment of heart failure, but now ACE inhibitors are accepted as the mainstay of therapy.

The single most frequent cause of hospitalization for persons sixty-five years of age or older is heart failure. About 400,000 new cases of heart failure are reported each year. However, despite the strongly favorable evidence and guidelines, ACE inhibitor therapy remains underused. Although ACE inhibitor therapy has been proved beneficial for congestive heart failure, less than one-third of patients who were candidates received this therapy. Widespread use of these therapies would profoundly change the health outcome for millions of patients who have had a heart attack and for those with congestive heart failure.

## Pain Medications (Analgesics)

Chronic pain has a major impact on quality of life and related disturbances in a person's feelings and behavior. For example, someone experiencing unrelieved pain may become depressed, even though the patient might deny pain. This possibility should be investigated if there is evidence of lethargy and sleep disturbance. In addition, chronic pain is usually coupled with social isolation and reduced ability to perform activities of daily living. These consequences are particularly important in older adults, who may rapidly become helpless and filled with despair.

Despite the importance of treating pain, medications are often underprescribed. In particular, nursing home residents with cognitive impairment tend to receive significantly less analgesic medication, both in number of drugs and in dosage, than their more cognitively intact peers. Analysis that statistically controls for the presence of painful conditions finds that doctors prescribe significantly less pain medicine for residents who are more disoriented and withdrawn. Likewise, nursing staff administer significantly less pain medication to residents who are more disoriented, withdrawn, and functionally impaired.

The same study revealed that health care providers lack knowledge about effective pain management in this population. Contributing to this lack of knowledge among providers is the medical field's limited understanding of how the nervous system processes painful sensory stimuli. Without a better understanding, health care providers are more apt to underrecognize, inadequately assess, and fail to treat pain in late life. For example, more research is needed to determine whether some patients express pain in more convincing ways, and whether some behave in ways that cause them to be viewed as overly dramatic, drug-seeking, or for some reason, undeserving of pain medication.

Among geriatric cancer patients, many experience pain daily yet receive no medication for pain relief. In an investigation of more than 13,000 cancer patients, medical professionals assessed the level and intensity of pain experienced by the patients, based on self-reports or, for patients who were unable to communicate, caregiver observation. The study found that 29 percent of the group experienced pain daily, and 26 percent of these patients received no treatment for relief of their pain. Moreover, 30 percent of those aged eighty-five years and older who reported pain went untreated, compared to 21 percent of those aged sixty-five to seventy-four. African-Americans had a 63 percent greater probability of receiving inadequate pain control than whites. Inadequate prescribing of pain medication is common among emergency department patients, and minorities are at higher risk than whites for undertreatment of pain.

In this study, the reasons for the differences in treatment included cultural and linguistic backgrounds and the patient's fear of becoming addicted to the pain medication. Furthermore, clinical training in pain management, other than for pain specialists, is almost nonexistent. Few health care professionals feel that they have received adequate training in pain management in medical school or during residency. Even those who have had specialty training in oncology report that their preparation for managing pain was inadequate. Clinicians are concerned that stronger analgesics may cause confusion, constipation, or balance problems. Although these concerns are legitimate, they do not justify undertreated pain. In addition, the aggressive use of controlled substances can raise fears of regulatory inquiry or the disapproval of professional colleagues.

Older adults facing surgery are a unique population. They may experience physical and mental limitation and may have different attitudes than younger patients when it comes to expressing pain and viewing the appropriate therapy for it. The altered physiology of aging changes the way the body distributes and metabolizes analgesic drugs and local anesthetics. These differences frequently require modifications in dosing and underline the importance of recognizing the unique features of geriatric patients in planning and providing pain medication before, during, and immediately following surgery. Single and combined therapeutic techniques that have been effective in younger adult patients are also effective (often with reduced drug doses) in geriatric patients without increasing side effects.

## Immunizations

Many older adults are not immunized against the serious diseases for which there are effective vaccines. Influenza and pneumococcal diseases are responsible for significant morbidity and for 50,000 to 80,000 deaths annually in the United States among high-risk populations and the elderly. Some high-risk populations are adults over sixty-five and those with diseases that increase their risk, including diabetes mellitus, chronic lung disease, and chronic cardiac disease. Other characteristics of underimmunized older adults are minority populations and those belonging to a low socioeconomic level or who are poorly educated and live in inner cities.

According to data from the Centers for Disease Control and Prevention (CDC), minorities have an especially low rate of being immunized for vaccine-preventable diseases. Some factors are recognized as reasons for the underutilization of vaccines in minority populations:

- Less access to care, related to low socioeconomic status and/or lack of health insurance for disease prevention and wellness
- Low incentive for primary-care providers to recommend and provide immunization to minorities because of low reimbursement rates
- Familial factors, such as lower education levels, poverty, language barriers, undocumented-immigrant status, inadequate knowledge of vaccine-preventable diseases, preconceived notions that vaccines are ineffective

Along with a relatively low level of vaccinations, providers of health care to minorities miss opportunities to perform tuberculin skin tests—for example, during office visits and hospitalizations. This is a serious oversight, since minorities are especially at risk for tuberculosis. One reason may be the relatively high proportion of foreign-born persons in certain minority groups. In 1996 the CDC reported that the incidence rate of tuberculosis among the foreign born was quadruple that of U.S.–born persons.

Within the United States, approximately 16 million Americans are infected with *Mycobacterium tuberculosis*. Individuals sixty-five years of age and older make up an estimated 25 percent of all active tuberculois (TB) cases. The vast majority of infected elderly are asymptomatic for TB yet harbor organisms likely acquired in the early part of the twentieth century. Of this group, 20 percent currently remain infected with the organism and account for the cases of TB disease in older persons.

For vaccination in general, some barriers to immunization are common within both healthy and high-risk groups:

- Skepticism about the effectiveness of the vaccine
- Uncertainty about side effects and adverse reactions
- Low concern for health, particularly among homeless, poor, or undocumented aliens
- Lack of physician contact
- Low recognition of the need for the vaccine (for example, the perception that the illness the vaccine protects against is minor)
- An attitude that immunization is inconvenient ("it's too far to go" or "there's not enough time")
- Cavalier attitude, as in "I don't need vaccines."

Professional medical organizations and national voluntary health organizations should expand outreach and develop policies to improve the rate and administration of influenza and pneumococcal vaccination among high-risk populations. These organizations should examine the emphasis among many health care providers on treatment of disease rather than on disease prevention. They also should improve immunization guidelines for high-risk populations. In addition, they should increase the gathering of data on the morbidity and mortality of vaccine-preventable disease in high-risk groups. Finally, the relevant organizations should develop a widely accepted standard of care for adult immunizations.

## Cost Control and the Expanding Role of Pharmacists

Critics of the health care industry have charged that in the United States, we spend as much to address the consequences of medication problems caused by inappropriate use of medications and the side effects of drugs as on the cost of providing the drugs in the first place. Pharmacists can help prevent such waste by monitoring the utilization of drugs, adverse reactions, and therapeutic failures. The American Society of Consultant Pharmacists has made some suggestions for controlling the cost of drug therapy and increasing patient awareness:

- *Generics*—Money could be saved by dispensing a generic version of an original-brand product, even though the original product is prescribed. Managed-care organizations and Medicaid programs often mandate the substitution of generics (except when substitution is specifically denied by the doctor).
- *Rebates*—Monetary incentives offered by pharmaceutical manufacturers to encourage increased use of their products. Mandated by federal law under Medicaid to ensure states of the discount prices that are available to other volume purchasers.
- *Unit of use*—The unit-of-use (unit dose) system was originally developed in hospitals and has since been adapted for use in most nursing facilities. This method provides a single dose of medication in an individual package, that can then be given to the patient without being "prepared" by a staff member. It can control costs and reduce the chances of medication errors by eliminating nursing staff preparation of doses.

- *Drug utilization review (DUR)*—This is a process that evaluates drug use, physician prescribing patterns, and patient drug utilization to determine appropriateness of therapy. Usually controlled by the state department of health.
- *Drug use evaluation (DUE)*—With DUE, health care organizations conduct a structured, ongoing, organizationally authorized quality-assurance process to ensure that drugs are used appropriately and effectively.
- *Drug regimen review*—A state review board of physicians, pharmacists, and nurses systematically evaluates medication therapy (reason prescribed, for whom, by whom) of resident-specific data. This type of review is beneficial because it can provide information about treatments that didn't work and drug side effects to health care professionals for future evaluation.
- *Patient counseling*—Physicians, nurses, and pharmacists should spend more time talking to patients about proper use, storage, and timing of drugs, as well as other aspects of using medications safely and effectively. Federal law requires this type of counseling in many inpatient and outpatient settings.

# Safeguards Against Inappropriate Prescriptions

In 1987 approximately 25 percent of noninstitutionalized elderly patients were taking prescription drugs that are widely regarded as unsuitable for their age group. Other drugs could provide the same therapeutic benefits with fewer side effects. This percentage would be even greater if it included potentially dangerous drug interactions or incorrect dosages. In 1992, 30 million noninstitutionalized Medicare recipients sixty-five or older used at least one drug identified as generally unsuitable for elderly patients, since safer alternatives exist. This represents 17.5 percent, an improvement over the 25 percent who used unsuitable drugs in 1987, but still a significant share of the population. Furthermore, the Food and Drug Administration (FDA) estimates that the annual cost of hospitalization due to inappropriate prescription drug use is more than $20 billion.

Federal and state initiatives have encouraged the development and dissemination of detailed information on the effect of prescription drugs on the elderly. The medical community has emphasized the need to increase physicians' knowledge of geriatrics and geriatric clinical pharmacology. The development of drug utilization review systems permits prescriptions to be screened *before* they are filled to identify potential problems. Finally, patients have become more proactive in their care. They seek information about drug therapies from several sources, such as consumer advocacy groups, state agencies, pharmaceutical companies, and the Internet.

Changes in the health care delivery system will help to reduce the inappropriate use of prescription drugs. Growth projections show that nearly one-third of all Medicare beneficiaries will be enrolled in managed care by 2009 (see Figure 4.1). Through utilization controls, managed-care plans have the opportunity to improve the coordination of drug therapies for newly enrolled elderly patients. Experts in the fields of gerontology and elderly clinical pharmacology, as well as representatives of the FDA and the Health Care Finance Administration (HCFA), have come together to investigate this situation. As a result, efforts to address the problem have been undertaken on the federal and state levels, in the medical community, and in the health care system.

The elderly, understandably, suffer from more illness and disability than do younger people. As a result, they account for a disproportionate amount of prescription drug use. While many prescribed drugs reduce illness and the risk of death in this age group, the balance between benefits and risks is precarious. As people age, there is a greater likelihood of adverse effects. This results from age-related factors such as changes in drug distribution in the body, in metabolism, in excretion, and in receptor sensitivity. If a practitioner is unaware of these factors, prescribing may be suboptimal, questionable, or inappropriate.

There is more than enough evidence to require ongoing, cooperative efforts to contain costs, identify appropriate geriatric pharmacologic interventions, and provide resources for clinicians charged with the responsibility of health care for the elderly.

# 5

# Sexuality of the Older Adult

IN U.S. SOCIETY, the usual perception among young and older adults is that elderly persons do not have sexual desires, are physically (therefore, sexually) unattractive, and are too fragile to engage in sexual activities. It therefore can be hard to acknowledge that aged persons participate in sexual activity. The media, families, and society in general view elders as deviant or ridiculous if they express sexual needs, desires, or behavior. Adult children dismiss the chance that their aging parents are or even could be sexually active. Despite these preconceptions, it is hard to explain why health professionals, who routinely ask pointed questions about other adult behaviors, neglect or overlook many of the sexual concerns of their geriatric patients.

Sexual desire and satisfaction are integral to human existence. Sexual adaptation is possible at any age among people who use the available resources. While the changes of aging affect sexual response in both men and women, aging does not eliminate the capacity to enjoy sex. For evidence of that enjoyment, watch elderly couples strolling the malls hand in hand, flirting among visitors to senior centers, and twin beds pushed together in nursing homes so the residents can still enjoy lying side by side.

The commonly held view that sexuality means intercourse is limiting. We can recognize many additional satisfying practices if we expand the definition of sexuality beyond intercourse to include touching, kissing, hugging, and hand-holding. In this broader context, although sexual intercourse may decline with age, a significant proportion of elderly persons remains sexually active.

# Influence of Aging on Sexual Function

The life expectancy in industrialized countries has increased, and the percentage of the population over the age of sixty-five tripled during the past century. As a result, understanding sexuality in the older adult and accepting that chronological age alone does not predict a person's sexual activity become vital. When sexual activity does decline, the cause is usually such factors as illness, drug interactions, lack of a partner, or negative perceptions of late-life sexuality.

Elders themselves can fall victim to the stereotype of the older adult as asexual. The stereotype thus creates a self-fulfilling prophecy of diminishing sexual activity based on low expectations, boredom with one's partner, or the false assumption that decline in performance is a normal part of the aging process. Furthermore, today's older adult has more conservative and restricted opinions of sexual attitudes than younger members of society. Such sentiments make it difficult for older persons to discuss sexual questions comfortably with clinicians. Nevertheless, research supports the view that satisfying sexual practices are possible at virtually any age.

With the proportion of the elderly population at 13 percent and growing, physicians will see significantly more older adults in their practices. Tending to their health needs will involve more than treating chronic debilitating conditions associated with aging. As people live longer, healthier, and more active lives, physicians will also need to address concerns about sexual health. The older adults themselves will need to recognize the significance of sexual health, and take steps to ensure it is not overshadowed by other physical conditions. Caregivers will need to understand that current stereotypical images of elderly sexuality are inaccurate and unjust.

# Common Myths About Older Adults and Sexuality

In our society, the prevailing ageist concept is that sexuality and physical attractiveness are attributes associated with youth. When caregivers or clinicians accept this concept and lack understanding of the older person's sexuality, they can make it difficult for the older adult to discuss sexual problems. Therefore, caregivers and health care professionals who learn more about aging and sexuality have important opportunities to help older persons improve the quality of their lives. That education may involve correcting some common myths about older adults and sexuality.

*Myth: "Old people aren't interested in sex."*

*Fact:* Decline in sexual activity has less to do with chronological age than with poor health, the unavailability of a partner, and the disapproving attitudes of adult children. Not only are older adults interested in sex, but they can enjoy sexual activity in many forms. In a study examining the sexual interests and behaviors of 80- to 102-year-olds, researchers found that 63 percent of men and 30 percent of women had remained sexually active. In addition, 72 percent of the men and 40 percent of the women engaged in masturbation. This widespread sexual activity reinforces the necessity of addressing social and psychological issues related to aging and sexuality in all areas. These issues range from masturbation to how to cope with the loss of privacy, especially when one or both partners reside in a long-term care facility.

*Myth: "Old people can't perform sexually."*

*Fact:* Aging is not synonymous with dysfunction. However, chronic illness and medication use—two factors that can impede normal sexual function—are more common within the older population than among younger adults. The major determinants of sexual activity for men are the ability to have erections, their overall health, and partner availability. Women's overall health and partner availability are equally important. Women's key physical challenge is coping with the decline in estrogen production, which causes reduced vaginal lubrication and loss of tissue strength and flexibility.

*Myth: "Sexual dysfunction in the elderly can't be treated."*

*Fact:* If the sexual problem is correctly diagnosed, treatment is usually possible. Available options include medications, prostheses, sexual assistive devices, and psychological counseling. Again, thorough and thoughtful medical evaluation is necessary to prevent myths from producing self-fulfilling prophecies such as problems with impotence because elderly persons think they are too old or unattractive for sex. Assessment of sexual problems has the added benefit of being an opportunity to detect early signs of other chronic disorders such as alcoholism, anemia, or diabetes.

*Myth: "Sex is only for the cognitively normal."*

*Fact:* Sexuality problems are certainly more complex for the cognitively impaired, and physicians who are treating patients with Alzheimer's or related dementias need to ask their patients' spouses about the entire range of sexual issues. Older adults may be embarrassed to discuss sexual problems, but when the discussion is in the context of the disease, the situation is more comfortable. Health professionals can also encourage alternative ways of expressing closeness and intimacy. For example, holding hands, massages, listening to music, and taking long walks together are ways of enjoying sensuality and intimacy that may otherwise be lost due to dementia. While long-term care does present certain problems, taking advantage of opportunities can offset many of them.

*Myth: "Old people don't get sexually transmitted diseases."*

*Fact:* According to a national survey of 14,000 people by the Center for AIDS Prevention in San Francisco, about 10 percent of a group of adults over fifty had one or more risk factors for HIV/ AIDS. The risk factors included multiple sex partners, a partner with a known risk factor, or a history of blood transfusions between 1977 and 1984. New AIDS cases are rising faster in middle-aged and older adults than in people under forty years of age, and 11 percent of all new AIDS cases involve people fifty and over. Most older adults who acquire HIV infections do so through sexual intercourse, and the disease is usually not discovered until it has advanced. In addition, older adults develop other sexually transmitted diseases besides HIV/AIDS. This further underscores the importance of clinicians taking a thorough sexual history when caring for their elderly patients.

*Myth: "Sexual identity is confirmed long before old age."*

*Fact:* Some researchers predict that health providers will see more older women involved in alternative lifestyles such as lesbian relationships, sharing partners, or asking for sexual advice previously associated with much younger individuals. These predictions are based on the increasing numbers of older women who outlive their spouses.

Many clinicians and social scientists dispute the idea of newly initiated lesbian relationships and partner sharing, but they agree that the significance of sexuality and the changes brought on by the uneven male/female ratio in the elderly population cannot be overlooked.

The interest in and happiness with sexual relationships remains strong in both hetero- and homosexual relationships. Most elderly gay men who are sexually active are satisfied with their partners and their sex lives. They report a positive sense of self-esteem, well-being, and contentment, and they generally have adapted fairly well to the aging process in terms of their sexuality. Other events that accompany aging, such as illness, reduced income, and loss of a long-term companion, cause the same emotional reactions among homosexuals as heterosexuals. However, negative social attitudes may make it difficult to find acknowledgment and support for their bereavement and grieving.

# The Aging Woman's Sexuality

The aging process is marked by a complex set of social, psychologic, and physiologic changes. All three components are important determinants of the sexual experiences of older adults. Of the older adult's experiences, a broad array, ranging from the act of sexual intercourse to a variety of feelings or emotions such as warmth or tenderness, belong in the category of sexuality.

Society's portrayal of the ideal sexual female as young, thin, and perfectly proportioned may be sexually inhibiting for an older woman dismayed by her aging body. Moreover, sexuality for both elderly women and men has long been described as inappropriate or, worse, an attempt to recapture youth. Even so, researchers have documented the importance of sexuality as a desirable, legitimate, and rewarding dimension of aging successfully. Expressions of tenderness and concern provide strength and positive motivation for all older adults.

Old age for many women involves many years spent as a widow. From the ages of sixty-five to sixty-nine, there are eighty-five men to every one hundred women. After the age of eighty-five, there are a mere forty men to every one hundred women. This female advantage in life expectancy, however, is offset by an increase in limiting chronic disorders, such as arthritis, incontinence, and hypertension. Because women live longer, they experience an increased rate of disability and a higher rate of institutionalization.

In addition to physical disability and availability of a partner, women's sexual activity varies according to social and cultural factors. And while sexual activity plays an important role in the lives of many elderly women through their seventies, eighties, and nineties, these older adults naturally undergo physiological changes that affect sexual functioning. Sexual interest and expression (libido) remain part of female behavior until advanced old age. However, expression of excitement can be delayed, with a reduction in vaginal lubrication, and the physical aspects of orgasm (vaginal and uterine contractions) can become less frequent. Other physical changes (identified in Table 5.1) begin at the time of menopause and slowly progress as a woman ages.

Female genital structures depend on estrogen, so the decrease in estrogen levels is responsible for the dramatic physical changes in aging female genitalia. Estrogen and progesterone levels, lower in older women than during their reproductive years, may affect female sexual behavior. However, we do not know the precise degree to which these hormonal changes influence sexual behavior. In one study of post-menopausal women, taking estrogen failed to influence the frequency of sexual intercourse or the intensity of sexual pleasure, although the estrogen did relieve vaginal dryness. Older women may therefore benefit from treatment with pills or creams. However, hormonal therapy has side effects, notably the potential for endometrial and breast cancer. Therefore, routine hormonal replacement is not advised solely for treatment of sexual dysfunction of older women.

Despite the physical changes associated with aging, health reasons alone are not enough to fully explain a decline in sexual activity and a rise in sexual disorders of the aged. Psychological and social factors also contribute to sexual disorders. Fortunately, changing attitudes of society have improved the understanding of the sexual needs of the aging population.

## Table 5.1 *Physical Changes in Elderly Females*

| Sexual Characteristic | Changes |
| --- | --- |
| Vagina | Epithelium thins<br>Vagina shortens and narrows<br>Vaginal acidity decreases<br>Risk of infection increases |
| Clitoris | Unchanged |
| Labia | Flattens and decreases in size |
| Pubic Hair | Hair thins<br>Distribution becomes sparse |
| Uterus | Size and weight decrease<br>Loses collagen and elastin<br>Glandular tissue declines<br>Interstitial fibrosis and sclerosis occur |
| Ovaries | Size and weight decline<br>Increased fibrosis and sclerosis |

# The Aging Man's Sexuality

Knowledge about the incidence of sexual dysfunction in elderly men is incomplete, because many of the elderly men who live with problems of this type do not seek medical help. As a result, the reported incidence of sexual issues of the elderly male is grossly underestimated. Sexual function is an important factor in the mental health and well-being of older adults, but health care professionals often overlook it. Why physicians and other practitioners fail to routinely assess geriatric sexuality is unclear. This oversight may be related to the sensitive nature of the topic, a lack of knowledge regarding sexual function in the aged, or the myth that the elderly are neither capable of nor interested in participating in sexual activity.

Men who are sexually active in their youth and middle years can remain sexually active in later life. However, several normal changes occur as men age. Men often notice the changes summarized in Table 5.2.

### Table 5.2 Physical Changes in Elderly Males

| Sexual Characteristic | Changes |
|---|---|
| Prostate | Size increases<br>Gland undergoes gradual enlargement<br>Gland may begin to block the flow of urine |
| Bladder | Wall thickens<br>Spontaneous contractions may occur when distended |
| Scrotum | Integument thins<br>Muscle tone declines |
| Testes | Size decreases<br>Firmness decreases |
| Penis | Wrinkling and hair loss<br>Dorsal vein may become visible |
| Pubic hair | Genital hair thins<br>Distribution becomes sparse |

Although the libido likely remains unchanged, men will probably notice that it takes longer to achieve erection, the erection may not be as firm, and it may take increased tactile stimulation to get fully aroused. The loss of erection after orgasm may be more rapid, and the force of ejaculation may not be as strong. Testosterone production decreases as men age. This decline is responsible for the diminution in size of the testicles and a decrease in sperm production. With aging, impotence seems to increase, especially among men with heart disease, hypertension, or diabetes. Many men can manage impotence, and in some situations, the condition can be reversed. It is important that men experiencing impotence share these concerns with their health care provider.

If either partner lacks understanding of these normal changes, anxiety increases and can contribute to additional sexual dysfunction. Disease, drug reactions, and disability also can contribute to emotional upset, decreased libido, erectile dysfunction, and inevitably, decreased sexual activity. Moreover, from a psychological viewpoint, men over the age of fifty must deal with one of the great fallacies of our culture: that every male in this age group is arbitrarily identified as sexually impaired. Together, these factors lead to a high incidence of sexual dysfunction in elderly men.

# Impact of Disease and Drugs on Sexuality

Many elderly adults are at risk of acquiring a chronic disease such as diabetes mellitus, hypertension, or emphysema. Such illnesses can precipitate changes in sexual behavior.

Older adults are frequently prescribed drugs that may interfere with sexual activity. Such drugs include antidepressants and antihypertensives. Older adults are also more apt to experience surgical procedures that can result in bodily disfiguration. Psychologic consequences may include diminishing or denying the older adult's sexual satisfaction. Examples of this type of surgery include prostatectomy in men and hysterectomy and mastectomy in women.

In addition to the problems caused by chronic illness, many disorders alter sexual activity by interfering with the blood supply or normal nerve functioning of the genitalia. Some of these common disorders are chronic prostatitis, cystitis, and urethritis. Also, incontinence (the inability to control the sphincters that govern urine and feces) causes alterations in sexual activity for both men and women.

Patients with a disability involving limited cardiovascular and pulmonary functions may have to avoid heavy exertion during sexual experiences. Clinicians can helpfully include suggestions for alternative sexual techniques when advising clients about their physical ailments.

> *Medical problems that may affect sexual functioning in men and women include heart disease, hypertension, arthritis, diabetes mellitus, Parkinson's disease, and chronic obstructive pulmonary disease.*
>
> *Psychosocial problems that affect sexual functioning include alcoholism, depression, stress and anxiety, and relationship conflicts.*

Alcohol use affects sexual function in both men and women. The depressant action of alcohol can cause erectile dysfunction in men and lack of libido in women.

Depression, anxiety, and chronic stress can interfere with the central nervous system pathways of sexual response. If the problem proves to be psychologic or psychiatric, the patient should be referred to a psychologist or psychiatrist for appropriate treatment and counseling. For example, men and women may experience dysfunction as a result of chronic disease or when concerned with their self-esteem. These situations require different treatment protocols from those designed to remedy depression. These factors need to be evaluated through a comprehensive interview and a physical examination, including laboratory data and investigative studies to determine the underlying etiology. The clinician's thoughtful attention in the treatment of sexual dysfunction in the elderly is critical, because simple reassurance often is enough to avert potential problems.

# Overcoming Sexual Dysfunction

Many problems with sexual dysfunction can be overcome, no matter what the person's age. The specific strategies may be as simple as education in technique or may involve changes in medication. The appropriate strategy depends on the source and type of dysfunction.

In the case of heart disease, if the disease is well controlled and treated, it is not necessarily a reason to abstain from having sex. The likelihood of a heart attack occurring during intercourse is extremely small. Four or five weeks after a coronary attack, if the patient can comfortably climb one or two flights of stairs or walk briskly around the block, the resumption of sexual activity is considered safe. However, patients have to be reassured of this by their physician before they resume sexual activity.

Patients with painful arthritis often benefit from teaching their partner to assume a different, more comfortable position. This strategy can prove to be mutually beneficial. Another way to improve sexual experiences for a person with arthritis is to coordinate it to take place during pain medication's peak effect.

Much of the sexual dysfunction in elderly persons is relatively easy to correct with general measures that can stimulate the libido and enhance the sexual experience:

- If a female partner is experiencing problems with vaginal dryness, substitute oil-based lubricants if water-based ones are ineffective.
- Initiate sexual activity when both partners are well rested.
- A hot bath promotes relaxation and enhances physical enjoyment.
- Erotic videos or literature stimulate some older couples.
- Decrease performance anxiety by not hurrying.
- Expand the use of touch and massage.
- Pay fastidious attention to personal hygiene.
- Practice Kegel exercises to improve muscle tone. Women are frequently told to do Kegels, but men also benefit, since these exercises improve muscle tone in both bladder and rectal areas.

### Table 5.3 Drugs That May Cause Sexual Dysfunction

| Classification | Drugs |
| --- | --- |
| Diuretics | Thiazide |
| Antihypertensives | Clonidine, reserpine, methyldopa |
| Major tranquilizers | Chlorpromazine, haloperidol |
| Minor tranquilizers | Pentobarbital, secobarbital, diazepam |
| Antidepressants | Nortriptyline, phenelzine |
| Miscellaneous | Alcohol, narcotics, nicotine |

Kegel exercises *involve contracting the muscles in the pelvic area governing urination and defecation. While sitting or standing, contract these muscles and hold for five seconds, then relax for ten seconds. Repeat for a total of five contractions. Do fifty a day.*

An elderly person with sexual dysfunction also might investigate whether medications are affecting libido and sexual performance. Table 5.3 lists commonly used drugs that may have such effects on men and women. Elderly persons taking these medications always benefit from discussing side effects with their doctor.

## Male Sexual Dysfunction

If medications are the cause of dysfunction in men, often the drugs can be changed or dosages modified. When the dysfunction is caused by a deficiency of the hormone testosterone, androgen therapy may be beneficial. However, such therapy is *not* appropriate for all older men. Androgens must be used with caution because they can stimulate growth of prostate tumors.

Other treatments may include the use of nonhormonal therapies including yohimbe (an herbal product) and topical nitroglycerin.

Another promising therapy for erectile dysfunction is sildenafil citrate (well known by its brand name, Viagra). Doctors and patients should consider that it has potentially dangerous interactions. It may *not* be taken by anyone also taking nitrates, a category of drugs used to treat heart disease. Some commonly used examples are: Nitro-Bid, Transderm-Nitro, and Nitro-Dur. Other drugs that interact with sildenafil include certain antifungal drugs and the antibiotic erythromycin. Other people who should not take sildenafil are those with preexisting cardiac risks or with impaired kidney or liver function.

Sildenafil citrate is taken orally, which tends to make it more appealing to men than alprostadil, another drug for erectile dysfunction, which is given by penile injection. Usually, the patient takes from 25 to 100 mg. of sildenafil one-half to four hours before sex. The drug suppresses levels of the enzyme phosphodiesterase, enabling the body to maintain high levels of cyclic guanosine monophosphate, which causes erections. This has been effective in many men with erectile dysfunction related to hypertension, coronary artery disease, psychogenic disorders, and to a lesser degree, diabetes and radical prostatectomy.

Following the release of sildenafil in 1998, there were reports of some fatalities and episodes of severe low blood pressure. Abnormally low blood pressure (hypotension) can be caused by a drug, an endocrine disorder, a neurological disorder, or a cardiac event (such as sudden irregular heart rhythm). The men who suffered fatalities related to Viagra had cardiac disease or were at high risk for it. Reporting complications and deaths from use of the drug is voluntary, and more clinical investigation into risk factors is needed. Another drawback is Viagra's high cost (as much as $10 a pill), although some insurance policies cover at least part of the cost.

Nevertheless, this therapy offers significant benefits. An unplanned benefit is that interest in Viagra is motivating more elderly males to seek medical treatment. Men in the fifty-plus age group tend to avoid routine medical checkups and to ignore the warning signals of disease. Doctors have found that about 30 percent of men who go to them complaining of erectile dysfunction also have undiagnosed conditions such as diabetes, hypertension, heart disease, or prostatic cancer. Perhaps the interest in Viagra will allow earlier detection and control of chronic disorders, thereby reducing morbidity and mortality and resulting in cost savings. Another potential benefit of sildenafil is that by extending the sex lives of middle-aged and older couples, it enhances well being and improves the quality of life for both partners.

For those who cannot take sildenafil citrate or prefer to avoid the risks, several alternatives are available:

- *Psychotherapy*—Patients often benefit from psychotherapy, regardless of the cause of sexual dysfunction. Working with a therapist offers the patient an opportunity to learn useful skills, which diminish anxiety related to intercourse.
- *Vacuum constriction device*—This consists of a plastic tube, which fits over the penis, and a pump that is used to remove air from the tube. Pumping air from the tube forces blood into the penis, which causes an erection.
- *Penile injection therapy*—A drug is injected into the side of the penis, where it works by dilating blood vessels and results in an erection.
- *Intraurethral therapy*—A soft pellet is inserted into the urethra, and the drug contained in the pellet is absorbed into the blood supply governing erection.
- *Surgery*—Surgical techniques include implants of prosthetics and/or vascular repair and reconstruction in the penis.

*The importance of a doctor conducting a thorough drug evaluation cannot be overemphasized. Some drugs cause impotence; others blunt libido or impair ejaculation.*

## Female Sexual Dysfunction

As a woman ages, an important biological factor is the decrease in the production of estrogen and androgen. These hormonal changes have a major influence on sexual response and often act to curtail it.

Traditionally, female sexual dysfunction has been treated with counseling and hormone therapy. The hormones estrogen and testosterone have been helpful in the treatment of some women. Hormone replacement therapy provides short-term benefits by improving over-all well-being and long-term benefits by enhancing cardiovascular and skeletal health.

Lack of estrogen causes vaginal tissue to atrophy, become dry, and easily irritated. Intercourse becomes painful, often resulting in minute fissures in the mucosa in the pelvis. Urinary tract infections can develop. The function of androgen is less clear. However, measured androgen deficiencies in older women are consistent with decreased libido, fatigue, and lack of well being.

In these situations, the use of estrogen replacement therapy relieves vaginal dryness and enhances sexuality—often eliminating the need for androgen replacement. The success of vasoconstrictive drug ther-apy for men may indicate a potential usefulness for women, while other products, which act by increasing blood flow to the genitalia are also being investigated for their potential.

A woman's diminished sexual response with age may be caused by painful intercourse (the technical term is *dyspareunia*), which occurs because of the aging process. As noted earlier, an aging woman's vagina shrinks and narrows, the vaginal epithelium thins, and lubrica-tion decreases. An effective treatment for these conditions is a vaginal estrogen preparation. However, such preparations are costly. If not cov-ered at least partially by insurance, this medication may be out of reach for elderly women on fixed incomes. In that situation, the application of an over-the-counter lubricant, such as KY jelly, before intercourse can effectively relieve symptoms of dryness. However, the lubricant will not retard vaginal atrophy.

Along with the physiologic changes affecting the sexual response of elderly women, attitudes and beliefs influence sexual behavior. Many older women have rigid viewpoints about what sexual activity is acceptable. Therefore, if conventional sexual intercourse is uncomfort-able or difficult for either partner, such women may reject alternatives.

# Sexuality After Surgery

The rate of recovery and return to sexual activity after surgery varies widely, depending on the type of surgery performed. Physicians and caregivers can enhance recovery and the return to previous levels of sexual activity by thoroughly explaining surgical procedures and by offering practical advice and emotional support before and after surgery.

Women tend to be less concerned about sexual performance than men, but they are more worried about their appearance. Men are more concerned about performance. However, elderly persons with cancer, for example, face unique challenges to their sexuality. Problems involve loss of body image, pain, hair loss, nausea, and vomiting.

Orthopedic and gynecologic surgery have their own significant recovery issues, ranging from the physical to the psychosocial and emotional. The patient may be dealing with pain, problems with mobility, fatigue, and, in the case of gynecological surgery, bladder spasms, fear of infection, and incontinence.

For help in coping with these issues, postoperative patients can participate in rehabilitation, support groups, and professional counseling. Postoperative success also depends on practical advice from health professionals as well as emotional support from the spouse or partner.

## Sexual Expression in Long-Term Care

Approximately 1.6 million persons live in about 20,000 nursing homes in the United States. Some residents are in a nursing home for less than six months, but the majority are in long-term care, living out their lives in the nursing home. Physicians, nurses, administrators, and other long-term health care providers need to offer a homelike atmosphere for these elderly persons.

Although sexuality is central to human behavior, it still may be overlooked by those charged with caring for nursing home residents. This population continues to have an interest in sexual expression. In spite of physiologic and anatomic changes, elderly men and women can continue to enjoy sexual experiences. When deprived of opportunities, they may engage in episodes of sexual acting out. Residents have been seen stripping off their clothing, touching other residents, or masturbating. While such behavior will gain the immediate attention of staff members, their reaction may be more punitive than constructive.

Researchers have surveyed nursing home residents and staff about their sexual beliefs. Results of the surveys indicate several barriers to sexuality among nursing home residents:

- Lack of privacy
- Chronic illness
- Staff attitudes
- Lack of a willing partner
- Loss of interest
- Feelings of being unattractive
- Personal lack of knowledge about sexuality

Lack of privacy is a common complaint among many nursing home residents. Nursing homes can surmount this barrier by allowing conjugal visits, using Do Not Disturb signs, or allowing doors to remain shut. Home visits could be arranged.

Chronic illness can interfere with sexual intercourse. The resident's doctor should assess the resident's medication regimen and investigate any dysfunctions produced by various disorders. A sexual history can give important direction to the individual's needs and desires, bearing in mind that there is more to sexuality than coitus. When the patient's doctor understands the problem, he or she can offer specific suggestions.

Staff attitudes vary widely. Some staff members infantilize elders who express affection for each other, referring to them as "cute." Others view the aged person's display of sexuality as deviant. Although these attitudes likely outweigh positive reactions to patient sexuality, there has been significant improvement in such areas as respecting the residents' rights to privacy.

Loss of interest and feelings of unattractiveness are closely related. Nursing home administrators can make beauty salons, barbers, and cosmetic services available for residents. Using these services improves the older adults' feelings of self-worth. Compliments by staff often boost residents' self-esteem.

Lack of a willing partner negates the lifelong need to share intimacy and to have that experience appreciated. Sexuality is part of one's identity, and if there is no one to share it with, the resident feels isolated. With guidance, the older adult can be encouraged to expand the meaning of sexuality to include pleasurable fantasy and attention to certain comforting feelings such as the soothing motion of rocking in a chair or music heard and perceived through vibrations. Nonthreatening touch such as handclasps or stroking of a pet also are calming and enjoyable.

A more difficult problem surfaces when a resident makes advances toward another who has dementia or is otherwise impaired. In such cases, staff must carefully evaluate each patient's decision-making capacity to prevent one resident from taking advantage of another. Similarly, care must be taken when the person *making* the advances has dementia. Psychiatric consultation is also helpful in evaluating these patients.

Residents who display inappropriate sexual behavior such as public masturbation require immediate and consistent intervention and redirection. Staff can be trained in basic behavioral therapy—for example, avoiding the reinforcement of unwanted behavior by overreacting.

## Safe and Healthy Sexuality in Long-Term Care

As the number of elderly nursing home residents increases, it becomes more important to ensure a homelike atmosphere. The residents' caregivers and doctors can help by encouraging privacy for residents and by educating staff about the changes of aging that affect sexual functioning. In addition, nursing home workers also need to recognize and encourage forms of sexual expression other than intercourse—for example, hand-holding, hugging, and touching.

With the current expansion of long-term care facilities, it becomes ever more important to stress that residents in geriatric settings should not be denied the kind of health advice on sexual issues that would routinely be given to much younger adults. In recent years, the most fruitful efforts to provide a clearer understanding of what is meant by sexuality and to explain the implications of the definition for health care have been the result of in-service education of staff by social workers and psychologists. In 1987 the World Health Organization set forth the following definitions of sexuality and sexual rights as follows:

- The capacity to enjoy and control sexual and reproductive behavior in accordance with a social and personal ethic
- Freedom from fear, shame, guilt, false beliefs, and other psychological factors inhibiting sexual expression and response
- Freedom from organic disorders, diseases, and deficiencies that interfere with sexual and reproductive function

Deeper levels of sexuality involving emotions and feelings can also be the focus of tension for health care providers. If the older adult's emphasis is less on sexual function and sexual orientation and more on such issues as comfort, respect, and companionship, discussions and attitudes about the relationship will require thoughtful attention from the caregiver. Entering old age without your life partner is very threatening and lonely. Some older people find support and companionship in a new relationship, occasionally with someone of the same sex. In the following example, Larry and Edith found companionship in spite of their dementia.

Larry, a former athletic coach, is eighty-four and vigorous. He wears his white hair in a crew cut, and his bright blue eyes look directly at you when he speaks. However, his dementia has robbed his speech of meaning. His vigor is now confined to continual, aimless pacing, and it is hard to get his attention. Larry no longer recognizes the adult daughter who assumed responsibility for him a year ago when his wife died. The daughter willingly took him into her home, but she was unable to monitor his frequent wandering or to manage his outbursts. Reluctantly, she admitted him to the memory impairment unit of a local nursing home.

Edith, seventy-seven years old, is another resident of the same unit. She has no family and rarely has a visitor. Not surprisingly, depression complicates her Alzheimer's disease. Edith has a very poor appetite, and it is a challenge to get her into the dining room.

When a staff member does manage to seat her at a table, the next hurdle is to coax her to eat something while she is there. A cloud of soft, white hair frames her sad, heart-shaped face. She stares expressionlessly until she sees Larry. Then she smiles and seems to relax.

Larry and Edith walk the halls of the unit, hand in hand, and they sit side by side for various activities. When they are together, Larry takes his medication without becoming belligerent. When in the dining room, they share a table, and Edith will eat at least half of her meal. The staff knows that they are a couple, and although neither resident has verbal communication skills, they communicate clearly to each other their need for touch, intimacy, and closeness.

As far back as 1974, Alex Comfort documented the fact that institutionalized patients are able to experience sexual pleasure. Nevertheless, many health care workers in nursing homes rigidly suppress demonstrations of sexuality between residents. The reasons are twofold: Staff are uncertain of the individual resident's ability to give truly informed consent. And the adult children of nursing home residents influence staff to discourage such behavior.

Despite the physical and psychological benefits of sexual contact, there are clear risks for abuse. Informed consent is important. By law and enforced through long-term care administrators, informed consent has three conditions:

- Absence of physical and psychological coercion
- Mental competence
- Awareness of risks and benefits

Physical coercion is fairly easy to monitor because of the open nature of the long-term care setting. Psychological coercion is more indirect. The resident's family and/or friends may be able to help staff members determine what behavior is an authentic choice.

Mental competence requires viewing the decision in the context in which it is made. A resident might be unable to give informed consent for medication or treatment, because the decision requires the resident to understand complex information. But the same resident might well be capable of giving informed consent to share a sexual relationship, because that decision is based more on experience.

Awareness of risks and benefits is less clear. The resident may not be able to foresee the major risk (psychological), which is the experience of yet another loss. A resident's partner could be transferred, discharged, or could die. However, the benefit of being able to confirm a state of feeling good, of being less lonely, is much more likely.

Sexuality in institutions, especially among older residents suffering dementia, is one of the most frequently discussed topics in gerontology. It is important to educate staff about sexuality in the aged and to advocate for the use of limited competency standards to assess residents' capabilities. More guidelines need to be developed so researchers can gather valid and reliable data, which will then give doctors and staff members dependable assessment tools. Based on this information, caregivers will be able to ensure residents' sexual rights.

## Attitudes of Staff and Families

Nursing home placement can signal the termination of sexual freedom for older adults. Other persons assist residents with personal care, and because of a national shortage of nurses and nurses' aides, they are often members of the opposite sex. Doors are unlocked, private rooms are scarce, and the beds are single beds. Married couples may be in different rooms, on different floors. (This may be appropriate placement depending on the level of care needed by the individual.)

Impediments to sexual freedom for the nursing home population can usually be attributed to staff and family members' lack of accurate knowledge about older adults' sexuality or negative attitudes about older adults' sexuality. For example, staff members may see displays of sexuality as disruptive and thus as problems to be managed. Adult children may disapprove of permitting residents' sexual expression and view the nursing home policy as too risky.

Even when staff and family have learned to accept older residents' sexuality, it is sometimes necessary to redirect patients' desires for intimacy and physical pleasure—a resident may display inappropriate sexual behavior or may experience sexual frustration. In these cases, nursing home personnel can employ a number of helpful measures:

- Provide more occasions for men and women to participate in activities together
- Provide more human touch when interacting with residents

- Increase the use of music
- Introduce pets in areas where they are accepted, to encourage stroking
- Use yarn, velvet, satin, fake fur, and other soft materials in activities programs
- Develop programs to help staff and families reduce their discomfort with resident behaviors and to examine attitudes toward residents' sexuality
- Create sexual education programs and discussion groups for staff, residents, and families in order to understand facts, acknowledge personal attitudes, and decrease overreactions to sexual expression in long-term care.

# Role of the Health Care Professional

Health care professionals can make a major contribution toward educating the elderly about sexual matters, including dispelling myths that older adults may believe. The primary-care physician can aid the elderly patient by recognizing sexuality as part of the patient's identity. Regular health histories should include questions about sexuality.

Physicians' assistants (PAs) and nurse-practitioners (NPs) are often collaborators with physicians as midlevel providers of health care for older adults. They provide routine care, do physical exams, and are responsible for disease management as well as management of acute episodes. Research shows that these providers perform effectively in the delivery of basic care.

Physicians' assistants are licensed to practice medicine with physician supervision. PAs practice in over sixty specialty fields, but more than half work in primary care.

Nurse-practitioners are registered nurses with advanced education, usually at the master's level. They have the clinical competency necessary to deliver primary care. NPs have specialties in areas such as pediatrics, geriatrics, and neonatology.

All health care providers can gain satisfaction by making their clients' lives more satisfying through guidance, education, and counseling. They can incorporate an awareness of sexual concerns into routine assessment questions. This provides them with opportunities to offer strategies and interventions to enhance well-being.

## Changing Views of Geriatric Sexuality

At one time, people associated sex almost exclusively with reproduction. Elderly persons had mixed feelings about their attitudes and the attitudes of clinicians when they discussed sexual problems. Today, however, research and clinical experience have generated changes in the assessment and prioritizing of sexual issues of older adults.

An understanding and acceptance of the normal changes in sexuality that accompany normal aging will give elderly persons a realistic assurance that they are not suffering from an affliction, something that should be treated as a medical problem. Just as it is normal *not* to have the strength and agility of youth in old age, alternatives and modifications of sexual behavior are available for older adults. Nongenital forms of sexuality are particularly important for those for whom sexual intercourse is neither possible nor desired because they lack partners, are disabled, or are in poor health. Hugging, fondling, kissing, and hand-holding all bring about an essential element of intimacy and closeness when sexual intercourse is impossible or involves risk.

Above all, elderly people and their caregivers must avoid believing that the aging process necessarily eliminates either the need or the satisfaction that physical intimacy provides.

# 6

# Mental Health and Mental Illness

OF THE MANY mental health disorders experienced by older adults, the two categories rated the most serious mental health problems in the United States by the National Institute of Mental Health (NIMH) are depression and Alzheimer's and related dementias. NIMH has targeted these diseases as essential areas for aggressive, expanded research.

## Depression

Nearly five million older adults suffer from serious, persistent depression. Research indicates that 40 percent of the geriatric patients with major depression also meet the criteria for anxiety, an emotional disorder related to several pathologies such as cardiovascular, pulmonary, and gastrointestinal disorders. Older adults with even mild depressive symptoms face an increased likelihood of becoming disabled and of having a decreased chance of recovery, regardless of age and sex.

Although depression occurs frequently in the elderly population, it often goes unrecognized or is overlooked. As a result, depression among the elderly often is untreated.

According to NIMH, 70 percent of untreated depressed elderly suicide victims saw their primary-care physicians within the month before
their deaths. This contact with physicians indicates that the doctors
are in a position to help depressed patients. It is therefore urgent that
physicians improve the detection and treatment of depression. Primary-
care health care providers are in a unique position to assess suicide risk
by evaluating elderly patients' functional status, depressive symptoms,
and physical health. Inquiring about a person's mood and spirits gives
the doctor insight into the patient's emotional state.

## Myths About Suicide

- A person who commits suicide rarely gives any
  warning.
- The decision to commit suicide is irreversible.
- Most elderly suicide victims live alone and are seldom
  in contact with their families.
- Talking with someone who is depressed can prompt
  suicidal action.

Clinical depression is a precursor of suicide. If the clinician has a
strong suspicion of depression, the physical examination should include
direct questioning about suicidal thoughts and plans. If a patient
expresses suicidal tendencies, the doctor should immediately have the
patient hospitalized and refer the patient to a psychiatrist.

The Centers for Disease Control and Prevention have identified
elderly suicide as a major public health problem. The suicide rate for
people over sixty-five began to escalate in 1980 and has climbed each
year since. While only 13 percent of the U.S. population is older than
sixty-five, this group accounts for 20 percent of all suicides. The highest rate is among elderly white males aged eighty-five and older and is
about six times the national average.

# Facts on Elderly Suicide

- Older adults are known for noncompliance with medical regimens. They often take too much or too little of their prescribed drugs, so a suicide attempt may look like an accident.
- Elders die from self-induced starvation and dehydration. It is often difficult to determine if an elder stopped eating because of advanced dementia, caregiver error, or intentionally.
- Fatal "accidents" of elders may be superficially investigated.
- It is accepted that old people die, so a sudden death may not be questioned.

## *Signs of Depression*

Depression is not a part of the natural aging process. Although aging consists of inevitable changes and losses, the normal emotional responses of grief and sorrow do not resemble the extreme, persistent sadness that typifies depression and interferes with a person's ability to carry on daily activities. As the table indicates, the symptoms of depression identified by NIMH are both emotional and physical.

Diagnosis of depression in the elderly differs from and is more difficult than diagnosing depression in younger adults. There are several reasons why:

- Patients as well as families and health care professionals are unsure about the vague, indistinct symptoms expressed by elderly individuals.
- The elderly client focuses on physical ailments, rather than on feelings.
- People associate many symptoms of depression with aging because less is expected of older adults after retirement.

Depression symptoms such as decreased social activity, decreased energy levels, and sleep disturbances are signs of depression that may develop after age sixty-five, but are often mistaken for typical elderly behavior.

- Like their elderly patients, many physicians concentrate on whatever chronic physical illness is present, and they often overlook depressive symptoms.
- If an elderly patient has dementia, the dementia can obscure the diagnosis of depression.

Depression occurs in every socioeconomic group, yet most people do not understand this illness. For example, it is pointless to say to a depressed person, "Cheer up," or, "You have nothing to worry about," or "Pull yourself together." Clinical depression, the term given to a group of mood disorders, is caused by a complex chemical imbalance in the brain. Neural circuits (the "wiring" of the brain) and neurotransmitters (chemicals necessary for nerve cell communication and the regulation of mood, behavior, and thinking) are impaired. Improved technology has shown brain images of patients with depression. In these people, the neural circuits do not function correctly, and there is a neurotransmitter imbalance. One of the best-known neurotransmitters is serotonin, a chemical in the brain that helps to transmit messages along the nervous system.

### Table 6.1 Symptoms of Depression

| Emotional Signs | Physical Signs |
| --- | --- |
| Nervousness | Sleeping more or less than usual |
| Guilt | Eating more or less than usual |
| Restlessness, irritability | Extreme fatigue |
| Feeling unloved | Persistent headaches, stomachaches |
| Despair, worthlessness | Chronic pain |
| Reduced enjoyment of formerly pleasurable experiences | |

Certain risk factors increase the likelihood of depression. Genetic and environmental risk factors include a family history of depression, a poor self-image, and low self-esteem.

## Causes of Depression

- Genetic risk, poor self-image, and low self-esteem
- Side effects of medications
- Other illnesses, such as stroke or cancer
- Life events, such as death of loved ones, financial losses, divorce

Elders most at risk for depression are unmarried women who have experienced much stress in their lives and have no social supports. In this high-risk population, researchers have considered serious chronic illnesses—stroke, cancer, and dementia—to be possible causes of depression. Clinicians believe that depression weakens the immune system, thereby predisposing the person to other illnesses.

*Depressed women over sixty-five are twice as likely as other elderly women to sustain a spinal fracture and 30 percent more apt to experience a nonspinal fracture. The reasons are unclear, but one possibility is a general decline in physical function. Earlier diagnosis and treatment of depression could reduce fracture-related morbidity and mortality.*

### Diagnosis and Treatment

The NIMH lists several goals of treatment for depression:

- Decreasing the symptoms
- Reducing the risk of relapse and recurrence

- Increasing the quality of life
- Improving medical health status
- Decreasing health care costs and reducing mortality

Treatment for depression should begin with a thorough physical examination by a physician. Such an evaluation would include a complete history of symptoms, questions about alcohol and drug use, and inquiries about other family members who may have had depressive illness. A key element of the assessment is a mental status examination to determine whether the depression has affected speech, thought patterns, or memory.

*When health care providers see patients with dementia or depression, they should rule out neglect and abuse. Because abuse can lead to depression, and because signs of abuse can mimic symptoms of depression, questions regarding abuse are now included on most medical history forms.*

Treatment depends on the result of the physician's evaluation. There are many effective medications available to treat depression. The development of new and better antidepressant drugs has provided useful chemical solutions to the regulation of depression. However, information regarding the treatment of the very old—the most rapidly increasing segment of the population—is scant, so clinical recommendations are derived from experience with younger adults.

Two of the most frequently prescribed and widely researched antidepressants have been nortriptyline and desipramine. These two drugs have fewer and more easily managed side effects. Antidepressants to avoid when treating elderly persons are amitriptyline and imipramine, as they cause a drop in blood pressure, which can lead to falls and fractures. Older adults are also likely to experience the cardiovascular and sedative side effects of these drugs.

Patients are more accepting of drugs that have fewer side effects and they are also apt to be more compliant with the medication regimen. Paroxitine (Paxil) and sertraline (Zoloft) are selective serotonin reuptake inhibitors (SSRIs), drugs that help to restore the neurotransmitter serotonin to normal levels. Because they work in a different manner than past antidepressants, they are often better tolerated and have better results. Two of the newest antidepressants are mirtazapine (Remeron) and venlafaxine (Effexor). They are in the tetracyclics category, which work by helping to restore both serotonin and norepinephrine. These dual-acting antidepressants often have higher rates of remission.

Newer research is taking place to evaluate the role of hormones in the development of depression and to determine whether hormone replacement therapy will be beneficial for elderly depressed patients.

*For the treatment of chronic depression, the latest research shows that in certain instances women are more apt to respond to sertraline and men to imipramine.*

Using medication to treat depression in elderly patients is a major challenge for several reasons:

- Significant improvement requires a much longer time period with older adults than with younger ones.
- The physician must carefully determine a drug dosage that will be therapeutic yet not toxic.
- Most elders are noncompliant with a drug regimen. The NIMH estimates that 70 percent of elderly patients do not take 25 to 50 percent of their medication.

Besides drugs, another treatment used in managing the depression of elderly patients is electroconvulsive therapy (ECT), which is used more often in depressed elderly because the response rates to antidepressant drugs in elders are lower than in younger adults. However, a significant drawback to using ECT in the elderly is the danger of seizure activity. Maintenance treatments of ECT and antidepressants need to be investigated carefully by both patients and caregivers because of such risk factors as confusion, cognitive deficits, and coexisting medical problems. The National Institute of Mental Health is an excellent resource.

Some psychosocial strategies, strategies that combine psychological and social aspects, are effective at treating depression. Effective strategies include cognitive-behavioral therapy and interpersonal therapy. Cognitive-behavioral therapy seeks to help a patient recognize and change negative thinking patterns that contribute to depression. Interpersonal therapy concentrates on effective interactions with other people in order to improve relationships, which in turn can reduce depressive symptoms. These interventions are used either alone or in combination with antidepressant medication. The evidence shows that with proper treatment, elders can enjoy substantial improvement in their emotional state and quality of life, as well as less incidence of recurring symptoms. In some situations, mutual support groups are helpful when combined with other treatments.

In the past few years, the use of herbs as a treatment alternative has provoked much interest. In Europe, Saint-John's-wort (*Hypericum perforatum*) is widely used to treat depression, but it has not achieved the same degree of acceptance in the United States. However, there is widespread interest in Saint-John's-wort in the United States, and three governmental agencies—NIMH, the National Center for Complementary and Alternative Medicine, and the Office of Dietary Supplements—have joined together to conduct studies of this herbal remedy.

*Caution: On February 10, 2000, the Food and Drug Administration issued a Public Health Advisory that Saint-John's-wort appears to affect an important metabolic pathway used by many drugs prescribed to treat conditions such as heart disease, depression, seizures, certain cancers, and rejection of transplants. Health care providers should alert their patients about these potential drug interactions, and patients should not take herbal supplements unless they confer with a physician or other health care provider.*

Individuals vary in their response to treatments for depression. If symptoms have not improved after several weeks, the patient should return to the physician to reassess the treatment plan.

## Special Situations

The treatment of depression is more complex when patients have other illnesses, including dementia, and when they live in a nursing home. There are conflicting reports about the effectiveness of drugs when older depressed adults have a coexisting illness. Some clinicians claim that such illnesses will diminish the drug response. Nevertheless, patients with other illnesses are entitled to as much consideration in treating their depression as any patient with a medical problem.

A nursing home admission confirms a person's loss of independence, and depression is a natural reaction to this disruptive change in lifestyle. There is a high prevalence of depression among today's 1.5 million nursing home residents. Further complicating this problem, depression often develops as a consequence of Alzheimer's disease, dementia, or Parkinson's disease, which are common diagnoses in the long-term care setting. In spite of these common contributors to depression in the nursing home, residents' depression frequently goes unrecognized. The resulting cost of untreated depression is high in terms of pain and suffering.

Several obstacles commonly stand in the way of the identification and treatment of depression in the long-term care setting:

- The staff is not capable of timely and appropriate interventions.
- The complex features of both depression and dementia make it difficult to distinguish one from the other.
- Insurance reimbursement and physicians' time constraints often hinder diagnosis and treatment.
- The number of trained personnel may be too small.

To improve the care of depressed nursing home residents, both licensed staff and nursing assistants need more training in identifying the behavioral indications of depression. Yet, until the problem of persistent understaffing is resolved, the skills learned in training programs will not be adequate to meet current needs. Since undiagnosed depression is so widespread in nursing homes, many of these facilities have instituted routine depression screening for their residents.

Distinguishing depression from dementia complicates the clinician's assessment of the patient. One consistent difference, though, is that patients with dementia try to answer questions, while depressed patients are withdrawn, apathetic, and passive. The pain and suffering of depression are unnecessarily great. Since treatment is known to be effective, third-party payers, such as insurance plans and Medicare, should cover diagnosis and treatment at a rate equal to that for other medical disorders.

## Getting the Appropriate Help

Many elders who need treatment for depression refuse referrals to mental health professionals because of a perceived stigma. In a 1998 survey, the National Mental Health Association revealed the following public attitudes and beliefs about depression:

- Among adults aged sixty-five and over, 68 percent knew little or nothing about depression.
- Only 58 percent of adults aged sixty-five or older believed that depression is a health problem.
- Depressed older adults are more likely than any other health group to "handle it themselves." Fewer than half seek help from a professional.

Many elders who need treatment flatly reject the idea that they are depressed. More barriers to the management of depression in older adults are the opinions of some older persons that they are too old to get help, the belief that asking for help is a sign of weakness, the belief that, with time, the depression will go away, and ageist attitudes of health care providers. Some health care providers do not listen carefully to old people, are cynical about a therapeutic benefit of treatment, and may believe that depression in old age is "normal."

Despite these challenges, elders and their caregivers need to know how to get the help they require. The first resource is usually the family physician, but clinics and health maintenance organizations also can provide treatment or refer patients to mental health specialists.

Included in the broad range of mental health specialists are psychiatrists, psychologists, family therapists, social workers, mental health counselors, and psychiatric nurses. Of these, only psychiatrists are physicians, so they are the only specialists who can prescribe antidepressant medication. The other mental health specialists often work with psychiatrists to ensure that their patients receive the necessary medications and counseling. In addition, many members of the clergy are trained to deal with emergencies or are able to recommend sources of appropriate help.

Other resources are community mental health centers, which usually provide treatment based on the patient's ability to pay, and hospital and university medical schools, where research centers that study and treat depression are located. In times of crisis, an emergency room physician at a hospital can provide temporary help and will direct the patient and caregiver to follow-up treatment, or if available and necessary, will admit the patient to a psychiatric ward in the hospital.

The National Institute of Mental Health recommends four necessary steps to ensure that depressed older adults have access to the mental health care they need:

1. Participation by health care providers in continuing education programs that will increase their skill in recognizing depression and referring patients to mental health specialists
2. Increased outreach and case identification in minority communities
3. Programs that train care providers, including nursing staff, in community and institutional settings to identify the behavioral signs and symptoms of depression
4. Communicating to mental health providers about the benefits of social service innovations such as adult day care and senior citizen programs

Clearly, elderly depressed patients merit a range of treatment options as their roles in life change, social supports dwindle, and chronic medical conditions increase. One of the most compelling reasons for seeking professional help is the fact that nearly 80 percent of clinically depressed people can be successfully treated. A thorough assessment by a mental health professional can determine effective strategies for treatment. Ignoring or denying the persistent sadness only leads to unnecessary suffering.

# Dementia

As defined in the *Merck Manual of Geriatrics*, dementia is a deterioration of intellectual function and other cognitive skills, leading to a decline in the ability to perform activities of daily living. Commonly, the patient has trouble learning new tasks, following complex directions, and retaining information. There may be difficulty with decision making and problems with orientation. Judgment is flawed, and social activities and relationships become impaired. These signs of dementia occur because brain cells become impaired. As the disease that causes the dementia advances, more brain functions are lost.

George, eighty-two years old, illustrates a case of moderate dementia. George was a popular neighbor in his town house complex, peopled mainly by elderly widows. He was cheerful, friendly, and best of all, was usually available to take a neighbor along for a ride to the supermarket.

His son frequently asked George to give up his car, because George had had several minor accidents in the past two years. His eyesight was poor, and his reaction time was unreliable. Twice George forgot where he put the car and had to take a cab to his son's office, but he always had an excuse. He would say things like, "It wasn't my fault," or, "They don't know how to park." The last conversation with his son ended in a heated exchange of words. That same afternoon, as George slowly backed out of the driveway, he hit a neighbor, sending her to the hospital with multiple fractures.

Dementia differs in frequency, causes, and treatment effectiveness among ethnic groups. The growth rate in dementia of minority elders is almost double that of elderly white Americans. Also, because minority elderly have lower incomes, poorer health, and lower life expectancy than white elderly, they are at risk for developing dementia earlier and in a more virulent form.

There are many causes of dementia. The following are among the most common:

- Side effects of medications
- Tumors
- Head injury
- Malnutrition
- Long-standing substance abuse
- General medical conditions

Families and caregivers need to know that careful investigation and screening are necessary so that they do not overlook conditions that are potentially treatable. The slow, almost imperceptible diminution of the power to think, to plan, or to remember is the condition most dreaded by older adults. Not only does a person lose the ability to understand and reason, but also the stricken individual is eventually robbed of distinguishing features of personality and behavior as the disorder advances.

Cognitive impairment associated with dementia is a major public health problem in terms of morbidity and mortality, quality of life, and health care costs. By some estimates, dementia costs $100 billion in lost productivity and direct care costs, exclusive of care provided by family caregivers. Cognitive impairment is responsible for half of nursing home admissions.

In spite of the prevalence of dementia in elderly persons, dementia is *not* a part of normal aging. No one, whether health care professional, family member, or patient, should assume that it is.

## Types of Dementia

Dementia has traditionally been classified as either Alzheimer's type or non-Alzheimer's type. The former accounts for nearly 60 percent of cases. Doctors should screen patients carefully to distinguish between the two types. Depressed patients, those who take multiple medications, or patients who are alcoholic, often are misdiagnosed as to the type of dementia they have. Consequently, they may not be properly treated.

### Table 6.2 Reversible and Irreversible Dementias

| Reversible | Irreversible |
| --- | --- |
| Drug toxicity | Alzheimer's disease |
| Dehydration | Brain trauma |
| Infection | Parkinson's disease |
| Malnutrition | Stroke |
| Vitamin deficiency | Alcoholism |

Many older adults display signs of cognitive decline that go unrecognized and untreated. In almost 20 percent of such cases, treatment could reverse the condition. Table 6.2 summarizes reversible and irreversible causes of dementia. Even for irreversible dementia, detecting it early enables patients and their families to prepare for the inevitable financial, medical, and legal challenges lying ahead.

## Challenges for Caregivers

Not only do few adults plan how they will take care of their elderly parents or spouses, but those already involved in a caregiving situation rarely anticipate changes in the patient's needs. The common coping strategy, to "take one day at a time," works while the situation remains stable or if the changes are gradual. Most people do not look for information about community services until faced with a sudden reversal in their loved one's health. After experiencing such an event, however, caregivers are more receptive to new information.

Caregivers of dementia patients, whether at home or in nursing home settings, experience a variety of physical and emotional pressures and strains. Dealing with disruptive behaviors, for example, is particularly stressful.

How can a caregiver reason with someone who is unable to process information? It can help to have some understanding of the elderly person's feelings. Imagine how frightening it must be not to know who you are or where you are. More terrifying still is to be unable to voice your fears logically to your caregiver, to have no orientation to time, place, and personal identity while the identity of those closest to you is steadily receding. That is the world of the dementia patient.

Understanding the cause of a disruptive behavior also can help the caregiver identify an appropriate response. Table 6.3 identifies behavioral problems that are common among dementia patients, along with possible causes of each behavior. The caregiver can try addressing the possible causes, to see if they help to alleviate the problem behavior.

For the caregiver, reactions to disruptive behavior run the gamut from simple annoyance to uncontrolled anger. At the same time, caregivers (especially family members) are also dealing with sorrow, confusion, denial, and final acceptance. Since the demented patient becomes dependent and unpredictable, and relationships change with the deterioration, caregivers should seek some type of training in handling a patient or loved one with dementia. The caregiver's response to inconsistent and inappropriate behavior caused by the continuing deterioration of the brain depends on many variables. These variables include personal health, support systems, and an understanding of the disease.

### Table 6.3 Common Behavioral Problems and Possible Causes

| Problem | Possible Causes |
|---|---|
| Agitation, excessive restlessness | Overstimulation by people or sounds; pain; constipation; hunger |
| Paranoia, suspicion | Social isolation of persons who live alone; confusing routine of hospital or nursing home; realization of loss of control |
| Wandering | Need for more exercise; difficulty finding the toilet |
| Depression | Reaction to increasing loss of independence; periods of clarity alternating with confusion |

Family caregiving is a common occurrence, but usually one person provides most of the hands-on care. Not surprisingly, the most frequently reported consequence of caregiving is restriction of leisure time. Although each primary caregiver manages with different skills, respite is critical for all caregivers. In the recommendations of the Alzheimer's Disease and Related Disorders Association, one of the first steps in reducing caregiver stress is to make all caregivers aware of available community resources.

## Alzheimer's Disease

In 1909 a German doctor named Alois Alzheimer discovered atypical changes in the brain tissue of a patient who died of an unusual mental illness. These changes consisted of neuritic plaques (dense deposits of protein) and neurofibrillary tangles (twisted fibers that build up inside neurons). These abnormal structures, seen in an autopsy, are the hallmarks of Alzheimer's disease.

Alzheimer's disease disrupts thought, memory, and language abilities. Its cause is unknown, and there is no cure. Alzheimer's disease is the most common cause of dementia in older adults, afflicting about 3 percent of elders aged sixty-five to seventy-four and more than half of those aged eighty-five and older. Despite its prevalence, Alzheimer's disease is not a normal part of aging.

Researchers think that genetic and environmental factors are responsible for more than half of the cases of Alzheimer's disease. British and Norwegian scientists investigated dietary influences and found elevated levels of homocystine (an amino acid) and low levels of folate in patients diagnosed with Alzheimer's disease. Folate, also called folic acid, is important in the development of the central nervous system (CNS) and may have a significant influence on sound CNS function throughout life. Other investigators are convinced that viruses can cause the changes in the brain tissue.

*Low levels of estrogen in postmenopausal women may be associated with the development of Alzheimer's disease.*

Information about risk factors is more certain. Known risk factors for Alzheimer's disease include age and family history. In addition, head injury, ministrokes, and low educational status are suspected risk factors.

Currently, an estimated four million Americans over sixty-five suffer from Alzheimer's disease. This devastating illness not only affects families and caregivers, but also places an enormous economic strain on society. The National Institute on Aging places the cost of caring for one person with advanced Alzheimer's disease at about $50,000 per year, whether the patient lives at home or in a nursing home. Since the disease can last up to twenty years, the overall costs to families and to society are exorbitant. The over-eighty-five age group is the fastest-growing segment of the population and the most ravaged by Alzheimer's disease. These facts underscore the urgent need to develop successful strategies to delay or prevent the onset of this disease, now termed a national health problem.

## Diagnosing Alzheimer's Disease

The first step in diagnosing Alzheimer's disease is to have a physician take a thorough medical history, perhaps questioning the person's family or friends, to learn about any difficulties in performing activities of daily living. In some cases, an episode of delirium—an acute state of confusion with or without hallucinations and agitation—may have been present in the patient's history before the eventual diagnosis of Alzheimer's disease or dementia.

To help rule out other possible disorders, blood, urine, and spinal fluid tests search for genetic markers associated with Alzheimer's and a specific protein linked to the disease. Brain imaging by means of computerized tomography (CT), magnetic resonance imaging (MRI), or positron emission tomography (PET) can indicate suspicious physical changes in the brain.

Also included in the diagnostic process are tests of memory, problem solving, counting, and language. A well-known standard test is the Folstein Mini-Mental State Examination, which consists of questions designed to evaluate memory and orientation. The doctor can also show the patient a few common, everyday objects and then ask the patient to identify them. Another task is asking the patient to repeat a sequence of words and numbers. Although the examination is brief, it aids in evaluating a patient's memory and helps the doctor estimate the level of cognition. Interviews with family members and with the affected person also aid the physician in determining cognitive function.

Patients with Alzheimer's disease show considerable variation in the clinical characteristics of the disease, including the age at which symptoms appear; the rate at which the disease progresses; the appearance of disturbances of mood, thought, perception, and behavior; the development of parkinsonian features; and the presence of a family history of Alzheimer's disease. Generally, though, the Alzheimer's disease patient initially displays mild symptoms such as having trouble remembering names or events. Gradually, simple math problems loom as huge stumbling blocks. The daily routine of getting up in the morning and getting dressed may take hours and even then may be incomplete (socks are forgotten, a sweater is inside out). These signs are seldom alarming, but as time passes, routine tasks such as personal grooming or signing one's name become major challenges that signal the patient or a family member to seek medical help.

The cases of William, Lilly, and Al provide three examples. William is a robust sixty-nine-year-old widower whose two sons are quite worried. He lived alone for several years and seemed to manage quite well. But for the past few months, his sons have noticed some troubling changes in his behavior. He seldom shaves, is generally unkempt, and continually discards his mail unread. When either of the sons offers to help him with financial matters or personal care, he becomes agitated, calls them "foolish," and says they are "looking for trouble" because he cannot see that there is a problem. William has no awareness of his disease, does not know his limitations, and refuses assistance because he has no perception that he needs help.

Lilly, seventy-four, is charming and soft-spoken. She and her husband enjoy bowling, attending the local senior center, and visiting with their grandchildren. To all outward appearances, they seem to be a healthy couple, happily enjoying their retirement. However, Lilly cannot make a cup of tea for herself. She doesn't know what to do with the kettle, and her husband has to watch her closely in the kitchen so she doesn't get hurt. Lilly has also wandered away from their small ranch house, so her husband installed sensors on all the doors to alert him to Lilly's unscheduled departures. Occasionally Lilly taps her head and jokes with her daughter about her "forgetter" being turned on—a deprecating reference to her unreliable memory. Unlike William, Lilly is sometimes aware she needs help, particularly when she is in a situation that demands memory and judgment.

Several years ago, Al, now fifty-five, founded a contracting business that has become extremely successful. Within the past few months, however, he has noticed increasing difficulty estimating jobs and keeping appointments. He has since taken his son into the business, and now he relies more and more on his son's judgment. Al posts reminders, lists, and Post-It notes to himself all over the house, in his home office, and in his truck. After exhaustive tests, he was recently diagnosed with Alzheimer's disease, and he understands fully what this means. Because he has such a high degree of awareness of his diagnosis, Al is at risk for experiencing reactive depression.

The first National Institutes of Health clinical trial aimed at preventing or delaying the onset of clinically diagnosed Alzheimer's disease in persons at risk—the Memory Impairment Study—started in March 1999. The study indicated that early-onset Alzheimer's disease (before age sixty) is influenced by heredity. The APOE gene has been identified as a link to the more common Alzheimer's disease seen in elderly individuals. A test for this gene, when used together with other tests, seems to be a useful tool for physicians who are diagnosing people with the symptoms of dementia. Discovery of these factors is promising and offers hope for more effective treatment of Alzheimer's disease.

The earlier an accurate diagnosis of Alzheimer's disease is made, the greater the opportunity to manage symptoms. An early, accurate diagnosis is especially important to patients and their families, because it helps them plan for the future and choose care options while the patient can still participate in making decisions.

## Treatment of Alzheimer's Disease

The course of Alzheimer's disease varies with each individual. As yet there is no known treatment that can halt its progress, although there are two drugs that hold some promise when administered in the early stages of the disease. Furthermore, in some cases, vitamin E seems to delay the advance of Alzheimer's disease. An advantage of using vitamin E is that it has no known drug interactions. However, you should inform your physician if you are taking vitamin E, since it can increase the risk of bleeding.

Patients and their families will have many weighty decisions to make. As they cope with the devastating news of the diagnosis, they should begin by planning in the following areas:

- Limiting or discontinuing driving
- Reviewing wills and estate plans of all concerned family members
- Drawing up a power of attorney for medical and financial decisions
- Developing advance directives and/or living wills
- Investigating options for long-term care
- Identifying support groups and social service agencies
- Identifying the patient's strengths and weaknesses and highlighting the unimpaired abilities

As the disease progresses, patients gradually need increased supervision and monitoring. The increased supervision is required to prevent wandering, to oversee finances, and to ensure physical safety. This intensifies the stress on the caregivers who are safeguarding their patients. These caregivers will need some form of respite, such as adult day care or regular visits by a home health aide with dementia experience. Patients may also require evaluation for depression at this stage of the disease.

Ways to relieve behavioral symptoms such as sleeplessness, wandering, and anxiety involve redirecting the behavior. Caregivers can occupy the patient with simple activities such as looking at pictures, listening to music or "white noise" such as sounds of the ocean, or receiving gentle hand massage. These interventions make patients more comfortable and lessen their stress, as well as the stress on their caregivers. These strategies, either alone or combined with appropriate medications, are also effective in the management of verbal and physical aggression, depression, and delusions.

The Food and Drug Administration has approved two medications for Alzheimer's disease. The first is tacrine hydrochloride (Cognex), approved in 1993. The second is donepezil hydrochloride (Aricept), approved in 1996. Aricept has less severe side effects than Cognex and is often used to treat mild to moderate symptoms of Alzheimer's disease in adults who can tolerate it. Nevertheless, the drug is limited. It does not stop or reverse the progression of Alzheimer's disease, and it seems to help only some patients for a period of time ranging from a few months to about two years.

Supplements may play a role in the treatment of Alzheimer's disease. The use of *Ginkgo biloba* extract and phosphatidylserine (PS) has been helpful for some individuals with memory impairment. Supplements should be taken only with the knowledge and approval of a health care provider.

A healthy diet is important during all stages of Alzheimer's disease. The Alzheimer's Disease, Education, and Referral Center counsels that while no special diets or nutritional supplements have yet been found to prevent or to reverse the disease, a balanced diet helps to maintain general good health.

Researchers are investigating treatments with the potential for preventing Alzheimer's disease, including estrogen-like compounds, anti-inflammatory agents, antioxidants, and drugs that target cell death. The pace of research is accelerating, combining the search for causes and effective treatments, as well as efforts to prevent onset of Alzheimer's disease.

Health care providers need to closely monitor Alzheimer's disease patients, to evaluate the progress of the disease and detect the development of any additional illnesses. Behavioral symptoms usually arise as the disease progresses. Wandering, anxiety, and hostility often can be treated with some combination of medication and behavioral interventions to keep the patient more comfortable.

People who are severely impaired by Alzheimer's disease become completely dependent on caregivers for feeding, bathing, toileting, and other basic functions. At this stage, families can become overwhelmed. They need support and assistance in making the decision whether to increase the help at home or to consider nursing home placement.

## Impact on Caregivers

As Alzheimer's disease steadily destroys a person's memory and judgment, the caregiver observes erratic behavior. The steady loss of cognitive power alters the patient's emotions and behaviors. Among the changes that occur, physical or verbal aggression, pacing, and scream-ing arise out of the patient's feelings of anger, frustration, fear, and depression. The bizarre behavior and the change in a loved one's per-sonality, coupled with the need to provide constant attention for years, are the major reasons for caregiver exhaustion and depression. These incidents take a devastating physical and emotional toll on caregivers as well as on families and friends.

Most primary caregivers are spouses who are older adults them-selves and who often have their own health problems. The next largest group are older daughters, who are usually employed and manag-ing their own families in addition to their caregiving responsibilities. Caregivers reach the limits of their capabilities and tolerance when incontinence and aggression develop, and this combination is often responsible for nursing home admission.

Caregivers of Alzheimer's and related dementia patients spend more time on caregiving tasks than do caregivers for persons with other types of illnesses. Predictably, the resulting stresses compromise their work and family relationships. Among the most successful ways to help these caregivers are peer support programs that link caregivers with trained volunteers who have had previous experience with demen-tia patients. Nevertheless, caregivers need programs and support ser-vices tailored to the daunting challenges that Alzheimer's disease caregivers face daily.

Some caregivers dealing with the pressure and stress associated with dementia care are particularly at risk. The risk is greatest for those who are male, lack relief from caregiving responsibilities, and have pre-existing illnesses, such as heart disease. The risks incurred are increased cholesterol levels and blood pressure and decreased immune function.

## Non-Alzheimer's Type Dementia

After Alzheimer's disease, the second leading cause of dementia is multi-infarct dementia (MID), which accounts for about 15 percent of all cognitive impairment. MIDs result from stroke damage. The onset is sudden, and the illness advances much more rapidly than Alzheimer's disease.

MID is the effect of cumulative tissue damage in the brain caused by transient ischemic attacks (TIAs), also called "ministrokes" or "small strokes," which often go unnoticed. A blocked or ruptured blood vessel deprives the brain of oxygen and nutrients, a process that causes brain tissue to die. The body parts governed by the damaged tissue reflect the various disabilities seen in stroke, such as impaired vision, slurred speech, varying degrees of paralysis, and cognitive impairment.

There are about 730,000 new stroke cases a year, and stroke is the nation's third leading cause of death, following heart disease and cancer. However, aspirin use has been significantly successful in treating patients with TIAs and, in many cases, MID.

*Dental x-rays have revealed calcification accumulation in neck arteries. Such blockage can cause strokes. Dentists are learning how to identify these preliminary findings so they may direct at-risk patients to appropriate medical follow-up.*

The National Stroke Association (NSA) lists the following symptoms of TIAs or ministrokes:

- Sudden numbness or weakness of face, arm, or leg, especially on one side of the body
- Sudden confusion and trouble speaking or understanding
- Sudden trouble seeing in one or both eyes
- Sudden trouble walking, dizziness, and loss of balance or coordination
- Sudden severe headache with no known cause

These symptoms are not necessarily dramatic. They can be brief, and people tend to overlook or ignore them. However, someone who experiences any of these signs should report them immediately to his or her physician.

The NSA also lists the following threats as potentially contributing to the likelihood of a stroke:

- Elevated blood pressure
- Smoking

- Excessive alcohol consumption
- Elevated cholesterol
- Diabetes
- Lack of exercise
- Family history of stroke

Besides stroke, another prominent cause of dementia is Parkinson's disease. Parkinson's is a neurologic deterioration marked by tremor, rigidity, and severe gait instability. Dementia occurs in 20 to 60 percent of the cases, progressing slowly as the disease develops. Patients with Parkinson's are also at high risk for depression.

## Alcoholism and Dementia

Dementia in older adults with a history of alcohol abuse can be caused by several factors, including Alzheimer's disease, vascular disease, or alcohol itself. Moreover, alcohol-related damage to nerve tissue may be related to as much as 25 percent of dementia seen in the elderly population. Since alcohol-related dementia is thought to be partly reversible with abstinence, its prognosis differs from that for Alzheimer's disease. Research efforts are developing criteria for differentiating the diagnoses of these two dementias.

Problem drinking can occur at any age, and family members are not always aware that a relative is alcoholic. Two common examples of alcoholism in older adults are lifelong heavy drinkers and those who begin to use alcohol to relieve unhappiness in their later lives.

*The incidence of epilepsy peaks after age sixty. The annual incidence of epileptic seizures rises dramatically in old age. Dementia and alcoholism are risk factors associated with late-onset epilepsy.*

Alcohol is both a drug and a depressant. It diminishes alertness, judgment, coordination, and reaction time. Drinking increases the risks of accidents, particularly falls and motor vehicle accidents.

Elderly alcoholics are different from younger alcoholics because they usually have a variety of concurrent medical disorders common to aging adults. They also display age-related changes that significantly affect their detoxification. They can decrease the amount of alcohol they drink yet still become intoxicated. The aging body reacts to alcohol in the following ways:

- Because of a reduction in body tissue mass, the available fluid volume for alcohol distribution is altered. This increases alcohol's potency.
- Because the filtration processes of the kidneys are delayed, alcohol spends more time in the body and does more damage.
- Because liver function is more easily arrested, detoxification is prolonged.

Over the long term, heavy drinking damages the brain and central nervous system. Other organs injured by alcoholism are the heart and the stomach. Furthermore, alcoholism causes disorientation and impairs memory, symptoms characteristic of Alzheimer's disease.

Ingestion of alcohol is especially hazardous when combined with prescription or over-the-counter drugs. Older adults are heavy drug consumers, and the combination of alcohol and drugs is a significant problem for that population. Drinking while consuming tranquilizers, analgesics, hypnotics, or antihistamines is not only dangerous but, on occasion, fatal. As we age, metabolism slows down, and the body's ability to absorb and dispose of alcohol and other drugs changes. The way drugs affect the body and the way the body manages drugs markedly alters drug tolerance in the elderly. Although many drugs are prescribed with warnings about drinking, elderly patients should discuss with a physician and pharmacist the possibility of drug and alcohol interactions, in order to avoid potentially lethal consequences.

Alcohol consumption can contribute to malnutrition as well. Alcohol contains calories but no nutrients and contributes nothing toward general health. Additionally, alcohol exacerbates an older adult's already reduced absorptive and metabolic processes, an action that also fosters malnutrition.

If an older adult's alcoholism is serious, the person's doctor should refer him or her to an appropriate treatment facility. Hospitalization is often needed to safely monitor detoxification, since the consequences of alcohol withdrawal are more severe in the elderly.

## Special Care Units

As the population ages, the techniques for caring for dementia patients in nursing homes become more specialized. Special care units (SCUs) are separate sections in nursing homes for residents with dementia. The past decade has witnessed an enormous growth in the number of SCUs in licensed nursing facilities; as of 1996, nearly one in four nursing homes had at least one organized unit or program specializing in dementia care.

For people with dementia, SCUs offer programs and environments that differ from those offered in a traditional nursing home setting. For example, effective dementia programs feature small-group activities arranged by functional or cognitive ability levels. Safe environments for dementia patients feature secured exits, smaller dining rooms, and indoor-outdoor areas for wandering. Many of these units offer single-occupancy rooms. Caregivers investigating SCUs should look for the following features:

- Training of staff in dementia care
- Separation between dementia and nondementia-impaired residents both in physical space and in social activities
- Reduction of the disruptive stimulation of noises such as radios and alarms
- Many simple, planned activities
- Management and (where appropriate) tolerance of what appears to be undesirable and inappropriate behaviors
- Participation of dementia residents in organized recreational activities

## Conclusions About Dementia

On the basis of ongoing research, the National Institute on Aging and the National Institutes of Health conclude that the dementias associated with aging are caused by more than seventy disorders and diseases that have overlapping characteristics and make accurate diagnosis difficult. Alzheimer's disease, however, probably accounts for more than 60 percent of all dementias and is the primary cause of institutionalization of elders over eighty-five years of age.

The cognitive impairments of aging have a far-reaching impact on economic and social resources and on society in general. In addition, the incidence of cognitive impairments and dementias profoundly affects households, as does the extent of institutionalization and health care expenditures. The shifting demographic and economic patterns among younger adults will determine what resources will be available in the future for caregiving.

# 7

# Elder Abuse and Ageism

THE IMPACT OF the expanding population of older adults is social, political, and economic. As a result, many public policies have been developed to meet the needs of these elders in the areas of retirement, health insurance, and long-term care. Nevertheless, in spite of these efforts, the abuse and neglect of the elderly who reside in their own homes is often overlooked and unreported. The important issues are recognizing the abused elder, identifying the perpetrator, providing effective interventions, and using prevention techniques.

## Recognizing Abuse

According to the National Elder Abuse Incidence Study of 1998, the different kinds of elder abuse and neglect are physical abuse, sexual abuse, and emotional or psychological abuse, with several subgroups in each category.

*Physical abuse* is the use of physical force that may result in bodily injury, physical pain, or impairment. Physical abuse may include such acts of violence as striking (with or without an object), hitting, beating, pushing, shoving, shaking, slapping, kicking, pinching, and burning. Other examples of physical abuse are the unjustified administration of drugs and physical restraints, force-feeding, and physical punishment of any kind. The following conditions may indicate that an older adult has sustained physical abuse:

- Bruises, black eyes, welts, lacerations
- Untreated injuries in various stages of healing
- Broken eyeglasses
- Signs of being restrained
- Older adult's report of being hit or mistreated
- Caregiver's refusal to allow visitors to see the older adult alone
- Laboratory findings of drug overdose or underutilization of prescribed drugs
- Broken bones
- Rope marks

*Sexual abuse* is nonconsensual sexual contact of any kind with a person. Sexual contact with any person incapable of giving consent also is considered sexual abuse. It includes unwanted touching, as well as all types of sexual assault or battery such as rape, sodomy, coerced nudity, and sexually explicit photographing. The following indications are warning signs of sexual abuse:

- Bruises around the breasts or genital area
- Unexplained sexually transmitted disease or genital infections
- Unexplained vaginal or anal bleeding
- Torn, stained, or bloody underclothing
- An elderly adult's report

*Emotional* or *psychological abuse* is the infliction of anguish, emotional pain, or distress on a person. Emotional or psychological abuse includes verbal assaults, insults, threats, intimidation, humiliation, and harassment. Also covered by this definition is the treatment of the older adult as an infant and the isolation of the older adult from family, friends, or regular activities. Additional examples of emotional or psychological abuse are giving an older person the "silent treatment" and enforcing social isolation. Older adults who are being emotionally or psychologically abused will seem either agitated or upset, or they may be very withdrawn and unresponsive. If they have the opportunity, they may even report this type of abuse themselves.

*Neglect* is defined as the refusal or failure to fulfill any part of a person's obligations or duties to an elderly adult. Neglect may also include a refusal or failure by a person who has fiduciary responsibilities to provide care for an elder (such as failure to pay for necessary home care service or the failure on the part of an in-home service provider to provide necessary care). Neglect typically means the refusal or failure to provide an elderly person with such life necessities as food, water, clothing, shelter, personal hygiene, medicine, comfort, personal safety, and other essentials included as a responsibility or an agreement. A neglected older adult will show signs such as the following:

- Dehydration, malnutrition, untreated bedsores, poor personal hygiene
- Being unattended or having untreated health problems
- Hazardous or unsafe living conditions (for example, improper wiring, no heat, and no running water)
- Unsanitary or unclean living conditions (for example, dirt, fleas, lice on the person, soiled bedding, fecal/urine smell, inadequate or inappropriate clothing)

Increasing numbers of men and women over the age of eighty and with cognitive deficits are found to be victims of many types of ill treatment. They are the group most at risk for abandonment, financial or material exploitation, and self-neglect.

*Abandonment* is the desertion of an elderly person by an individual who has assumed responsibility for providing care or by someone who has physical custody of an elderly person. Elders have been abandoned when they are admitted to a hospital, nursing home, or similar setting. Frail, cognitively impaired older adults have been recovered after they were deserted in shopping malls, bus terminals, or other public locations. Occasionally, an older adult is able to self-report abandonment.

*Financial* or *material exploitation* is the illegal or improper use of an elder's funds, property, or assets. Some typical examples include cashing checks without authorization or permission, forging an older person's signature, misusing or stealing an older person's money or possessions, coercing or deceiving an older person into signing a document (for example, contracts or a will), and the improper use of conservatorship, guardianship, or power of attorney. Elderly persons are targets for unscrupulous individuals who gain their trust and then proceed to exploit the elder financially or materially. The following evidence is consistent with indications of financial or material exploitation of an older adult:

- Sudden changes in a bank account or banking practice, including unexplained withdrawals of large sums of money by a person accompanying the elderly person
- Unauthorized withdrawal of funds using an elder's ATM card
- Abrupt changes in a will or in other financial documents
- Unexplained disappearance of funds or valuable possessions
- Charges for services that are not necessary
- Discovery of an elder's signature forged for financial transactions or for the titles of the elder's possessions
- Sudden appearance of previously uninvolved relatives claiming rights to an elder's affairs and possessions
- Unexplained sudden transfer of assets to a family member or someone outside the family

*Self-neglect* is characterized as the behaviors of an elderly person that threaten the person's own health or safety. Self-neglect generally manifests itself in an older person's refusal or failure to provide him- or herself with adequate food, water, clothing, shelter, safety, personal hygiene, and necessary medication. The definition of self-neglect, however, does not apply in a situation where a mentally competent older person makes a conscious and voluntary decision to engage in acts that threaten personal health or safety. The following are cardinal signs of self-neglect:

- Dehydration, malnutrition, untreated or improperly attended medical conditions, and poor personal hygiene
- Hazardous or unsafe living conditions (for example, improper wiring, no indoor plumbing, no heat, and no running water)

- Unsanitary or unclean living quarters (for example, animal or insect infestation, no functioning toilet, fecal/urine odor)
- Inappropriate or inadequate clothing
- Grossly inadequate housing or homelessness

# Who Are the Abused?

The National Elder Abuse Incidence Study gives evidence as to the violence and neglect experienced by the elderly. The study estimates that at least one-half million older adults suffer from physical abuse or neglect and that for every documented occurrence, about five are unreported.

Researchers have outlined several risk factors: problems of the abuser (substance abuse or mental illness), financial dependency of the abuser on the older adult, social isolation, and stress. Elderly widows who live with a troubled, dependent child are frequent victims. The child is usually in need of housing and money, and the mother is too intimidated and ashamed to do anything about the situation.

Female elders are abused at a higher rate than males, even allowing for their larger representation in the aging population. The oldest old (eighty years and over) are abused and neglected at two to three times their proportion of the elderly population. In almost 90 percent of the elder abuse and neglect incidents with a known perpetrator, the abuser is a family member. Two-thirds of the perpetrators are the victims' adult children or spouses. The victims of self-neglect are usually depressed, confused, or extremely frail.

When Irene, eighty-four, was brought to the emergency department by her daughter, she was malnourished, dehydrated, and barely conscious. Her hair was matted, her nails were long and dirty, and she smelled of urine. There was a bedsore on her sacrum and several bruises on her extremities. When questioned, the daughter said that her mother had a poor appetite, and she didn't know what fluids her mother consumed, since she (the daughter) was gone all day. She did say that her mother spent most of her time in bed "resting" and was often incontinent.

After a week of careful evaluation and systematic, aggressive treatment, Irene was stable enough to respond to questions from a social worker. She stated that she lived with her daughter, a fifty-five-year-old waitress, who was frequently unemployed. She denied that the daughter caused the bruises found on her extremities, yet when the daughter visited her, Irene clearly seemed to be afraid of her. The daughter's visits were infrequent, but when she did show up, the nursing staff detected the odor of alcohol on her breath. While it was never determined that Irene was physically abused by her daughter, she was clearly a victim of neglect.

Sixty- to seventy-year-olds make up almost 70 percent of elders being physically abused, although they represent only about 45 percent of the elderly population. Among adults eighty and over, neglect is the most frequent type of mistreatment.

Although elder abuse is seen in all races and ethnic populations, most of the reported incidents involve victims who are white. In four out of five categories of elder abuse, white perpetrators outnumber all other racial/ethnic groups. (The white population is also dominant, so these statistics reflect the general population.) However, full documentation of elder abuse in immigrant populations is scarce, mainly because of language barriers and cultural practices.

Irene fit the major criteria for elder abuse:

- She was female.
- She was over the age of eighty.
- Her abuser was a known family member.

Irene was eventually admitted to a local nursing home with the unwritten direction to all nursing personnel to "monitor for potential abuse." A staff member was directed to be nearby whenever the daughter visited so Irene's safety was ensured. Many long-term care facilities employ this simple, effective strategy if a visitor potentially could jeopardize a resident's safety or well-being.

## Influence of Physical and Mental Impairments

Elderly people with physical and mental frailties are more likely to be vulnerable to abusive behavior. About 15 percent of older adults in the United States are depressed at one time, 10 percent suffer from some form of dementia, and nearly 14 percent have difficulties with one or more activities of daily living (bathing, toileting, dressing, etc.). While rates of depression remain fairly stable across the life span, physical and mental impairments increase, especially after the age of eighty-five.

The data indicate that a large proportion—about three out of four—of elderly abuse and neglect victims are physically frail. Irene, the eighty-four-year-old abuse victim, was not only incontinent, but she also was probably too weak and unsteady to get out of bed to go to the bathroom to toilet herself.

# Who Are the Abusers?

An analysis of documented incidents of elder abuse indicates that men were responsible for 52.5 percent of the occurrences, with the remaining 47.5 percent caused by women. Neglect is the only type of abuse committed with nearly equal frequency by men and women. Financial/material exploitation is the second most commonly found maltreatment, with men accounting for close to 60 percent of perpetrators. Emotional/psychological abuse was the third most frequent type of abuse. Just over one-half of those responsible in this category are male. Of those who abandon older adults, 83 percent are male.

The majority of abusers of elderly persons are concentrated in two age groups: those aged forty and younger (adult children) and those older than age eighty (spouses).

Among the known perpetrators of abuse and neglect, the abuser was a family member in 90 percent of the cases. Two-thirds of the abusers were adult children or spouses. Flora's story and Ernie's story provide two examples of typical situations.

Flora, eighty-two, had Parkinson's disease and was a resident in a nursing home. She lived in the home for four years while her illness advanced to the point where she could do very little for herself. Flora's Social Security check went directly to the nursing home, which deposited $40 into her account for personal shopping. This amount usually paid for her weekly beauty shop appointments in the home and birthday cards for grandchildren, with a little left over for occasional clothing items.

Flora's account rapidly dwindled to a balance of less than $60, and the nursing home's social worker discreetly questioned her. It turned out that Flora's fifty-year-old daughter was regularly "borrowing" money. "But she's going to pay me back soon," Flora claimed. Since she denied there was a problem, there was little the administration could do. The money was never repaid.

Ernie's situation is similar, but had long-term effects. When Ernie's wife of fifty-one years died, he remained in the small ranch house that they had paid off together. Ernie, eighty-five, felt comfortable there. He lived on his modest pension, and for emergencies he had a nest egg accumulated over his years of owning a small business. He thought he was fortunate, despite his chronic emphysema and failing eyesight. Ernie's son, a forty-eight-year-old with an erratic work history, offered to help his father pay bills, balance his checkbook, and manage his money.

Soon the son began to coax Ernie to invest in a vague, "surefire" stock that a friend "guaranteed" would yield an enormous return on his investment. The son was persistent, mentioning how it was a once-in-a-lifetime opportunity for Ernie to build a comfortable estate for himself, his son, and two grandchildren. He repeatedly appealed to Ernie's affection for the grandchildren. Eventually, Ernie relented and entrusted the entire nest egg, $80,000, to his son. The stock failed, the lucrative returns never developed, and the loss of his savings plunged Ernie into a deep depression.

Researchers investigating spousal abuse found that the demands of caregiving were not necessarily predictors of violence. However, the age of the caregiver was a risk. The older the spousal caregiver, the more likely the incidence of domestic violence. Moreover, many men who customarily abused their wives still abused them as they grew old.

# Self-Neglect

The term *self-neglect* refers to the conduct of an older adult, generally one who is living alone, that threatens his or her own health or safety. In such situations, the older adult refuses to provide him- or herself with available means to ensure physical health and well-being. In documented incidents of self-neglect, approximately two-thirds of self-neglecting elders are female.

In a midsized city in New England, an elderly man was found frozen to death after several days of bitter cold weather. Although the man lived alone, he had a family who knew that his heating system was not functioning. They had tried to help, but he rejected their offers of assistance. He flatly refused to let anyone come in to fix his furnace, saying that he would take care of it himself. Neighbors had warned him and tried to help. They also met with abrupt refusal. That was in the fall. When he finally did get around to calling the appropriate repair service, he did not convey the urgency of the problem, and he was put on a waiting list. A sudden, unexpected cold spell in mid-November accompanied by a freak snowstorm caused the indoor temperatures to plummet. The eighty-year-old man crawled into bed and tried to warm himself with blankets, but the weather was too severe, and he died of hypothermia.

Perhaps this tragedy could have been averted. But there are individual differences to honor and barriers to overcome. For example, legal mediation may be impeded under the following circumstances:

- An individual is competent, so intervention that is not requested may not be feasible.
- Agencies must respect religious and/or cultural traditions, even though some may appear to be onerous and contribute to self-neglect.
- Long-standing self-neglecting behavior is frequently paired with an unrecognized mental health disorder. As these individuals age, physical and cognitive impairments exacerbate the mental health problem. If the mental health problem remains unrecognized, legal mediation threatens to jeopardize patients' rights and civil liberties.

The largest proportion of self-neglecting elders (45 percent) are in the oldest age category—those eighty and older. The older an elderly person gets, the more likely it is that he or she will be self-neglecting. Over three-quarters (77.4 percent) are white, and another 20.9 percent are black.

A common reason for self-neglect is difficulty caring for oneself. Among older adults with verified self-neglect, 93 percent have some difficulty caring for themselves. Another contributing factor is some degree of confusion.

# Abuse as a Threat to Life

In August 1998, the *Journal of the American Medical Association* described a study that was the first to compare mortality of people who have been mistreated to that of their nonvictimized counterparts. The study, which took place at Yale University and was funded by the National Institute on Aging (NIA), yielded research data on nearly 3,000 adults over sixty-five, with an average age of seventy-four. The population studied was divided into three parts:

- Those whom another person had referred to protective services for mistreatment, including abuse, neglect, or exploitation
- Those who required protective services for self-neglect
- Those who had no referral to protective services

The researchers found that at any time during the follow-up period, people seen for maltreatment or self-neglect had, overall, a poorer survival rate and an increased risk of death. Abused elderly had a 3.1 times greater risk of dying than did those with no reported mistreatment. The risk for the self-neglected was 11.7 times greater. This increase in risk takes into account factors associated with death in older people, such as dementia, depression, chronic disease, functional problems, and socioeconomic status.

NIA scientists stated that the Yale study's findings are an important step in understanding and preventing abuse of older people. Further research will cover risk factors leading to abuse and neglect, such as family dynamics, and the consequences of abuse and neglect in addition to death, such as decline in general health status and problems with family interactions.

# Reporting and Preventing Elder Abuse

Four types of gatekeeper agencies are charged with identifying elder abuse and neglect:

1. Law enforcement departments
2. Hospitals and public health departments
3. Banks
4. Elder care providers

In cases of self-neglect, the most frequent reporters of confirmed observations of this abuse are hospitals and friends or neighbors. Family members of victims report 20 percent of cases of elder abuse and neglect, followed by hospitals (17 percent) and police departments (11 percent). Other sources that report are churches, apartment managers, fire departments, landlords, residential facilities, utility companies, and anonymous reporters.

If you observe evidence of elder abuse or neglect, call the Area Agency on Aging (AAA) listed in the state or federal government section of the telephone directory (usually under "aging" or "elderly services"). This agency can determine who has jurisdiction over the geographical area where the older adult lives. If you cannot locate the number or are unsure of which office has jurisdiction over the area in which the older person lives, call the Eldercare Locator at 1-800-677-1116. This hot line functions from 9:00 A.M. until 8:00 P.M. Eastern time, Monday through Friday, with voice mail taking messages after those hours. It is sponsored by the Administration on Aging. When you call, be prepared with the address of the older adult's residence, including the zip code.

## *Prevention of Elder Abuse*

State legislatures in all fifty states have passed laws (for example, elder abuse, adult protective services, domestic violence laws, mental health commitment laws) that authorize the state to protect and provide services to vulnerable, incapacitated, or disabled adults.

In more than three-quarters of the states, the services are provided through the state social service department (adult protective services). In the remaining states, the State Units on Aging have the major responsibility. Agencies screen calls for potential gravity. Some states operate hot lines twenty-four hours a day, seven days a week. The agency keeps information received in reports of suspected abuse confidential. If maltreatment is suspected, an investigation is conducted (in cases of emergency, usually within twenty-four hours). On the basis of a comprehensive assessment, a care plan is developed which might involve one or more of the following actions:

- Obtaining a medical assessment of the victim
- Admitting the victim to the hospital
- Helping the victim obtain needed food, heat, or medication
- Arranging for home health care or housekeeping services
- Calling the police
- Referring the case to the prosecuting attorney

Once the immediate situation has been addressed, the appropriate adult protective services (APS) agency continues to monitor the victim's situation and works with other community agencies serving the elderly to provide ongoing case management and service delivery. However, an older adult has the right to refuse services offered by APS unless the court declares the adult incapacitated and has a guardian appointed.

If a concerned citizen or a practicing professional who serves the elderly suspects that abuse has occurred or is occurring to an older adult known to the individual, these suspicions may be reported to the local APS agency. Most states require certain professionals to report abuse. (If the suspected incident involves an older person living in an institutional setting, the call should be placed to the office of the local long-term care ombudsman, described in Chapter 8).

To obtain the telephone number for the APS office, call directory assistance and request the number for the department of social services or aging services. To reach a long-term care ombudsman, call the Area Agency on Aging, which is listed in the government section of the telephone directory under "aging" or "elderly services."

# The Older Americans Act and the Administration on Aging

Older adults and their caregivers should learn the relationship between the Older Americans Act (OAA) and the Administration on Aging (AOA). The OAA of 1965 established the AOA, which is an agency of the U.S. Department of Health and Human Services. The Administration on Aging has the following priorities:

- Building systems of home and community-based long-term care
- Promoting consumer empowerment and protection
- Serving as a focal point for information and education about aging

Several titles of the Older Americans Act provide for supportive in-home and community-based services. For example, Title III supports a range of services, including nutrition, transportation, senior centers, homemaker services, and health promotion. Title VII emphasizes elder rights programs (including the nursing home ombudsman program), legal services, insurance counseling, elder abuse prevention efforts, and outreach. Under Title VI the AOA awards funds to 216 tribes and native organizations to meet the needs of older American Indians, Aleuts, Eskimos, and Hawaiians. The grantees provide services in keeping with the unique cultural heritage of these Native Americans.

Program funding is allocated to each state Agency on Aging based on the population of elderly persons. Some 660 Area Agencies on Aging receive funds from their respective state agencies. The Area Agencies on Aging contract with public or private groups to provide services such as the following:

- *Access services*, such as information and referral, outreach, case management, escort and transportation
- *In-home services*, including chores, homemakers, personal care, home-delivered meals, and home repair and rehabilitation

- *Community services*, such as senior centers, congregate
  meals, adult day care, nursing home ombudsmen, and elder
  abuse prevention
- *Caregiver services*, such as respite care, counseling, and
  education programs

Older adults, their caregivers, and anyone else concerned about the
welfare of an older person can contact the local Area Agency on Aging
for information and referral to services and benefits in their community. These agencies are usually listed in the Yellow Pages under city or
county government headings. Also, a nationwide toll-free hot line, the
Eldercare Locator provides information about assistance for older
adults anywhere in the nation. The number is 1-800-677-1116. Callers
must provide the elder's address, including zip code.

## State Elder Abuse Prevention Programs

In general, states have focused their elder abuse activities in four areas:

1. *Professional training*, including skill-building workshops for
   adult protective services personnel, designed to introduce
   specific professional groups such as law enforcement, to
   aging and elder abuse issues; statewide conferences open
   to all service providers with an interest in elder abuse; and
   development of training manuals, videos, and other materials
2. *Coordination among state service systems and service
   providers*, such as creating elder abuse hot lines for reporting; formation of statewide coalitions and task forces; and
   creation of local multidisciplinary teams, coalitions, and task
   forces
3. *Technical assistance*, which may involve the development
   of policy manuals and protocols that outline appropriate
   procedures
4. *Public education*, for example, development of appropriate
   elder abuse curricula for elementary and secondary school
   students; development and delivery of elder abuse prevention
   public education campaigns, including radio and television

public service announcements, posters, flyers, and videos with training materials suitable for use with community groups

# Why Does Elder Abuse Occur?

Elder abuse, like other types of domestic violence, is extremely complex. Generally, a combination of psychological, social, and economic factors, along with the mental and physical conditions of the victim and the perpetrator, contribute to the occurrence of elder maltreatment. Each incident and each type of abuse involve a variety of causes, so a short list of factors cannot explain all types of elder maltreatment. However, the following list describes some of the predominant causes that researchers have identified:

- *Caregiver stress*—Caring for frail elderly people is very difficult and stressful. This is especially true when the elderly charge is mentally or physically impaired, when the caregiver is poorly prepared for the responsibility, or when the necessary resources are lacking. Under these circumstances, the increased stress and frustration of a caregiver may lead to abuse or willful neglect.
- *Impairment of the dependent elder*—Many researchers have found that elders in poor health are more likely to be abused than those in good health. Abuse tends to occur when the stress level of the caregiver is heightened as a result of the older adult's worsening cognitive or physical impairment.
- *Cycle of violence*—Violence is a learned behavior, and it is transmitted from one generation to another. As a result, some families are more prone to violence than others. In such families, abusive behavior is the normal response to tension or conflict because family members have not learned any other ways to respond.
- *Personal problems of abusers*—Abusers of the elderly (typically adult children) tend to have more personal problems than do nonabusers. Adult children who abuse their parents

frequently suffer from mental or emotional disorders, alcoholism, substance abuse, relationship problems, and financial difficulties. Because of problems like these, the adult children often depend on the elders for their support. Abuse in these cases may be a grossly inappropriate response by the adult children to a realization of their own inadequacies.

> *Caregivers who have difficulty coping with the demands and obligations of caring for an older adult may use alcohol or drugs as a misguided coping mechanism.*

# Protecting Residents of Nursing Homes

Residents of nursing homes and other long-term care facilities have the right to reside in a safe and secure environment and to be free from abuse and neglect. Title 42, Code of Federal Regulations 483.156, requires the states to establish and maintain a registry of nurses' aides that includes information on "any finding by the State survey agency of abuse, neglect, or misappropriation of property by the individual" involving the elderly.

The National Child Protection Act, as amended by the Violent Crime Control and Law Enforcement Act of 1994, encourages the states to conduct national background checks of job applicants. However, federal law does not require criminal background checks of current or prospective employees of federally assisted long-term care facilities or a registry for staff other than certified nursing assistants who work in these facilities.

While there is no federal requirement for criminal background checks, most states require such checks, either by law or by regulation. Nevertheless, states' requirements are widely divergent. For example, there is no uniformity in designating the facilities and the personnel covered, establishing the systems used for the check, determining the use of state or federal records or both, fingerprinting requirements, the types of crimes that disqualify a person from employment, the factors determining suitability for employment, or the assignment of costs and payments for the criminal background check.

There is no standard protocol for the states that do have criminal background checks. Some require background checks for certified nursing assistants (CNAs) applying for jobs, but do not include current employees or other personnel such as owners, nurses, dietitians, and housekeeping staff. Most states do not include staff currently employed, contractor staff, or volunteers. The sources for the background checks vary widely. State or FBI records may be used either combined or separately. States have indicated certain crimes that would automatically disqualify some applicants, but the disqualifying crimes vary from state to state.

In a 1998 audit, the Office of the Inspector General, Department of Health and Human Services, queried thirty-seven states as to the types of registries maintained that supplied pertinent information. According to the audit report, titled *Safeguarding Long Term Care Residents*, all thirty-seven states had registries for certified nursing assistants, licensed practical nurses, registered nurses, and medical practitioners, even though federal regulations mandate only the CNA registry. The audit also provided the following data from registry officials:

- 94 percent do not initiate criminal background checks on applicants when they apply for certification or licensure.
- 29 percent do not require information of prior arrest or conviction on the renewal application.
- 13 percent do not provide for a penalty for making false statements on the certification or license application.
- Convictions for crimes committed outside of the long-term care facilities are not systematically reported to the registry.

Regulations of the Health Care Financing Administration require that the nurse's aide registry of each state include information on convictions for elder abuse and on findings of abuse, neglect, or misappropriation of property. This information is stored permanently in the registry unless it is found to be erroneous, the individual was found not guilty in a court of law, or the individual dies. Furthermore, nurs-

ing facilities must report to the state nurse's aide registry or to licensing authorities any knowledge they have of court actions against an
employee that would indicate unfitness for service as a nurse's aide or
other facility staff.

Criminal background checks offer long-term care facilities an
important opportunity to help safeguard against hiring persons who
ever abused or neglected vulnerable elderly residents. Anyone with
questions regarding the policies for background checks in their own
state's long-term care facilities should begin their investigation by calling the Eldercare Locator at (800) 677-1116.

# Ageism

Ageism is a prejudice against older adults expressed through attitudes
and behavior. Age discrimination may be obvious, such as a television
station replacing a seasoned, fortyish news anchor with a pretty,
though inexperienced, young woman. Yet it is the subtle form of age
discrimination that can have the most powerful effect in shrinking or
terminating an employee's productive years. For example, in the movie
and television industries, twenty-something executives pass over the
older, experienced writers with proven track records in favor of writers in their own age range. In less prominent business areas, a new,
young manager can make life so uncomfortable for his sixtyish inher-
ited office assistant that eventually the assistant will leave.

Stories like Tracy's abound. Tracy, a fifty-eight-year-old nurse edu-
cator with two masters' degrees, retired from her fifteen-year career
as the dean of a nursing program in a local community college. Her
husband had retired two years earlier, and after much thought, they
decided to move to a warm, southern state to pursue their fondness for
golf. After several months, Tracy became restless, so she answered an
ad for an adjunct professor in a local university nursing program. She
neither wanted nor needed tenure track. Although her clinical skills
and teaching credentials were current and impressive, the college hired
a young woman with a baccalaureate degree and no teaching experience, who had been out of college less than four years.

Age discrimination is sometimes allowed to continue with little protest because of a long-held assumption that it is right and appropriate for older workers to step aside to make room for younger workers who need to support families. This pattern was developed and fostered during the Great Depression of the early 1930s. Now, however, low unemployment characterizes the economy. Many older workers want to work to share their experience and skills, but frequently the mature employee is working because the supplemental income is needed.

Employees take advantage of retirement at age sixty-two or earlier in response to ageism and a combination of several issues:

- A negative work climate that favors younger employees
- The desire for independence
- The belief that Social Security or a pension plus savings will provide living expenses
- Ignorance and fear of rapidly changing technology

Ageism may play a larger part in the decision than most people are willing to admit. Older workers are often viewed as being less competent and not worth training for jobs.

Financial need and career interests send many early retirees back to work. Working elderly pay more for retirement, pension, and Social Security contributions than do nonworking elderly across all income levels. Also, regardless of income level, nonworking elderly spend more on health care than do working elderly.

In the last decade, downsizing, increased use of part-time and contract workers, greater reliance on automation, and less job security in general have created what may be regarded as an atmosphere of expendability. In such a climate, it is the older worker who is at particular risk of losing a job. Several years ago, the American Association of Retired Persons (AARP) published a report titled *American Business and Older Workers: A Road Map to the 21st Century*. According to personnel directors and company executives interviewed for the AARP report, older workers rated very highly, but these managers believe younger managers "do not really want older employees," no matter how good their skills. Many of the decision makers said that younger managers see older workers in the following terms:

- As "Mom and Dad," so they do not want to boss them
- As knowing more than baby boomers do, which makes younger managers look bad (less competent)
- As hard to relate to, not part of the younger manager's generation
- As "inflexible, unwilling to change"

## Age Discrimination in Employment Act (ADEA)

In 1967 Congress enacted the Age Discrimination in Employment Act (ADEA) to prevent employment discrimination against workers aged forty and over. Under the ADEA, an employer may not discharge, refuse to hire, or otherwise discriminate on the basis of age in compensation, terms, conditions, or privileges of employment. The ADEA requires that ability, not age, determine an individual's qualifications for getting and keeping a job. The ADEA protects individuals who are forty and older. It applies to job applicants as well as employees, but it does not apply to elected officials or independent contractors.

The ADEA also helps employers and employees find ways to resolve problems that arise from an aging workforce. If an employee is unable to resolve the matter of perceived age discrimination, he or she has the right to file a charge with the Equal Employment Opportunity Commission (EEOC). (The EEOC also handles complaints about discrimination against employees or applicants on the basis of race, color, religion, sex, national origin, or disability.) A person who files a complaint, participates in an investigation of an EEOC complaint, or opposes an employment practice made illegal under any of the statutes enforced by EEOC is protected from retaliation.

The EEOC investigates charges that are filed, but it dismisses many complaints. Litigation is costly both financially and emotionally. It is also time consuming. The older adult deciding whether to pursue a discrimination charge must weigh the positive and negative aspects carefully. For advice and direction, examine the home page of the EEOC's website, www.eeoc.gov, or telephone the agency at 1-800-669-EEOC.

Older workers are stable and responsible employees. Their work ethic makes them valuable recruits for employers.

## *General Legal Assistance*

In many states, special statewide legal hot lines are available to help with a range of legal and related problems. This innovative delivery system provides both quality assistance for simple issues and referrals when more extensive help is needed.

## *Pension Counseling Programs*

Many people are confused by the technical language and numerous contract provisions associated with their pension plans, and they are intimidated by the procedures in pursuing claims. The Administration on Aging funds a Technical Assistance Project at the Pension Rights Center in Washington, D.C., as well as six demonstration projects around the country. All of these projects have the following objectives:

- Conduct outreach to workers confused about pensions
- Provide people with information and expert advice on pursuing claims
- Establish a system for referral of workers with complex claims to lawyers willing to help free of charge or at a reduced rate
- Encourage workers to take responsibility for their own income security in old age by understanding their pension plans

For further information, call the Administration on Aging's Eldercare Locator at 1-800-677-1116 between 9:00 A.M. and 8:00 P.M. Eastern time, Monday through Friday. Voice mail will take a message after the stated hours.

# 8

# Long-Term Care

LONG-TERM CARE embraces a continuum of health, social, and residential services devoted to meeting the needs of impaired persons. Most clients of long-term care facilities are elderly. Currently there is an active trend toward change in how long-term care is delivered and paid for. The urgency of the movement is emphasized by the fact that the expense of long-term care—especially nursing home care—can rapidly deplete a family's resources.

Many Americans assume that Medicare or their traditional health insurance will cover the costs of long-term care. Too often it is only when a family member becomes disabled that they learn of their responsibility for the expenses. When the need for long-term care develops suddenly, families are poorly prepared to determine what types of services will be in their best interests. In many circumstances, $100 a day is a modest outlay for care in the home. Institutionalized care can easily surpass $70,000 annually. These obligations can bankrupt even middle- and upper-middle-class families.

Despite often heroic efforts by family members to care for older family members at home and help pay for uncovered expenses, many elderly and disabled persons ultimately rely on Medicaid to pay for their long-term care. Medicaid has become the primary payer of long-term care costs. In 1997 the Health Care Financing Administration (HCFA) reported that nursing home costs and home care costs exceeded $69 billion. For many states, the costs of long-term care consume most of the state budgets, and the sobering reality is that these costs will continue to grow as the population ages. Both federal and state governments acknowledge a compelling need to control the ever-expanding costs of long-term care, yet neither the public nor private sectors have found adequate ways to finance them.

As we saw in Chapter 1, the percentage of Americans sixty-five and older has more than tripled, and the older population is living longer. These trends have serious implications. Long-term care has become increasingly significant because its costs absorb much of the budget available for health care for all ages.

Most older adults are independent, but with advancing years, particularly after the age of eighty-five, many elders need assistance with everyday activities such as bathing, dressing, shopping, cooking, and housecleaning. Limitations on activities due to chronic conditions increase with age. In a survey conducted in 1994 and 1995, more than half of the older population (52.5 percent) reported having at least one disability, and one-third of this group reported being severely limited by a serious chronic condition. The percentages of disabilities increase sharply with age, and these infirmities take a heavy toll on the elderly, both physically and financially. In 1997 older adults averaged $2,855 in out-of-pocket health care expenditures, a 35 percent increase since 1990.

# Preparing for Health Problems

In its 1996 report, titled *Aging into the 21st Century*, the National Aging Information Center documented projections of self-reported health status. About 10 percent of the elderly reported themselves to be in poor health in 1990. Blacks reported poor health almost twice as often as whites and others. Also, as age increased, more and more elders identified their health as fair to poor.

Health care emergencies such as a stroke or a fractured hip may propel elderly individuals and their families into hurried decisions. To avoid this pressure, older adults should investigate services before there is a crisis. Knowing what is available and affordable provides a measure of control for elders accustomed to being independent and in charge of their own lives. Furthermore, this is a constructive way to reassure families.

# What Is Long-Term Care?

The phrase *long-term care* spans a range of options that extends from temporary help to residential placement for people who have lost some capacity for self-care. Temporary help consists of aid offered by family members and friends and scheduled visits from a home health aide. Placement in a skilled nursing facility—either temporarily or permanently—provides an older adult with rehabilitation and skilled care twenty-four hours a day.

The choices for long-term care have never been more abundant. Services can include adult day care, transportation services, foster care, assisted living, and retirement communities, as well as traditional nursing homes. If support from family, friends, local meal programs, and transportation options become inadequate, the impaired older adult may need to move to a setting where care is available around the clock.

Frequently, the cognitive impairments and chronic diseases associated with aging limit what an elderly individual can do. When such impairments progress to the point where independent living is neither safe nor practical, residential placement is an alternative to consider. There are two types of residential settings:

1. *Assisted living*—This type of living arrangement can be set up as a "board and care" home for a small number of people, or it may be a large apartment complex or a building similar to a hotel or condominium. The levels of care offered vary but usually include meals, recreation, security, and help with bathing, dressing, medication, and housekeeping.
2. *Skilled nursing facilities*—Nursing homes provide twenty-four-hour services and supervision. The residents, who are generally frail, afflicted with many chronic diseases and in various stages of dementia, receive comprehensive medical care and rehabilitation where appropriate.

A variation of the skilled nursing facility is the continuing-care community. Health care providers offer different levels of care at one location, allowing a less disruptive transition from one type of care to another when it becomes necessary. Most have useful programs for couples, meeting the needs of both spouses when one requires more care than the other.

# Planning for Successful Long-Term Care

The National Institute on Aging recommends a four-pronged approach to planning for long-term care:

1. *Ask questions.* Doctors, friends, relatives, local hospital discharge planners, social workers, and religious organizations can provide information about specific facilities. Each state's Office of the Long-Term Care Ombudsman has information about specific nursing homes and any problems associated with that facility. Understand that other types of residential arrangements, such as board-and-care homes, are not required to follow the same federal, state, or local licensing regulations as nursing homes.
2. *Call.* Telephone places that seem appropriate. Ask basic questions about vacancies, the number of residents, charges and methods of payment, and Medicare and Medicaid participation. Determine convenience of location, transportation resources, meal provision, housekeeping options, activities, dementia units, and medication policies.
3. *Visit.* Make an appointment to visit various residences. Speak with staff, residents, and families of residents. It is also helpful to go unannounced and at different times of the day. Observe whether residents are treated respectfully. Is the building clean and safe? Sample the food.
4. *Understand.* When making a decision of this importance, get professional help in comprehending financial agreements and contracts from social service groups or attorneys specializing in elder law.

*Insurance coverage varies widely. The federal Medicare program and private Medigap insurance offer short-term home health and nursing home benefits. State-operated Medicaid programs can supply information about long-term nursing home coverage for people with limited means. Private long-term care policies are complex and costly. For further information, contact your state's insurance commission, listed in the state government section of the telephone directory.*

# Paying for Long-Term Care

Most people pay for long-term care with some combination of Medicare, Medigap plans, and Medicaid. These three resources are interrelated, yet distinct.

## *Medicare*

The federal government created Medicare to serve as a health insurance program for people sixty-five years of age and older, people with end-stage renal disease requiring dialysis or transplant surgery, and some people with disabilities. Medicare has two parts: *Part A* is hospital insurance, and most people do not have to pay for this element. *Part B* is medical insurance, and most people pay monthly for this coverage.

The original Medicare plan is available everywhere in the United States. It is the way most people receive their Part A and Part B benefits. An eligible individual may go to any physician, specialist, or hospital that accepts Medicare. Medicare pays part of the bill, and the individual is responsible for the remainder. However, some health care expenses are not covered by Medicare. For example, Medicare does *not* pay for the following expenses:

- Routine eye care
- Dental care

- Most prescription drugs
- Most chiropractic care
- Acupuncture

Table 8.1 provides more details about the extent of Medicare coverage, or you can call 1-800-842-2052 for complete Medicare coverage information.

In some parts of the United States, eligible persons may choose a Medicare managed-care plan, which is similar to a health maintenance organization (HMO). Participants in a Medicare managed-care plan may go only to a physician, specialist, or hospital that is part of the plan. Plans must cover all Medicare Part A and Part B benefits. Some of these plans cover extras, like prescription drugs. Out-of-pocket costs may be lower than in the original Medicare plan.

### Table 8.1  What Medicare Does and Does Not Pay For

| Required Charges for Medicare Services | Services Covered in Part by Medicare | Services *Not* Covered by Medicare |
|---|---|---|
| Part A deductible for each benefit period | Home health care that does not meet certain required conditions | Outpatient prescription drugs |
| Part B deductible of $100 per year | Cost for skilled nursing facility care for days 21–100 in the benefit period | Eyeglasses |
| 20% coinsurance for most Part B covered services | First three pints of blood needed each year | Hearing aids |
| | | Routine physical exams |
| | | Emergency care outside the United States |
| | | Custodial care |
| | | Orthopedic shoes for non-diabetics |
| | | Cosmetic surgery |
| | | Dental care |
| | | Dentures |
| | | Routine foot care |

A new Medicare health care choice available in some parts of the country is private fee-for-service plans. Individuals who enroll in such a plan may go to any physician, specialist, or hospital. Plans must cover all Medicare Part A and B benefits. The plan, not Medicare, decides how much the individual pays.

## Medigap Insurance

Medigap insurance plans are optional medical reimbursement policies, issued by private companies, which are designed to reimburse policy-holders for many of the medical expenses not covered by Medicare. As with all insurance contracts, plan benefits and premium costs for these policies vary among insurance companies and must be evaluated care-fully by the prospective buyer before purchase. As happens too often, holders of medical reimbursement plans are not completely aware of what their benefits are until after they have submitted a claim.

A reasonable amount of comparison shopping and product assess-ment is prudent before any final decision is reached as to what com-pany and plan provides the services needed.

## Medicaid

Medicaid, or Title XIX of the Social Security Act, is a program that provides medical assistance for individuals and families of any age with low incomes and inadequate resources. The Medicaid program became law in 1965 as a jointly funded cooperative venture between federal and state governments to assist states in providing adequate medical care to eligible needy persons. Medicaid is the largest program pro-viding medical and health-related services to America's poorest peo-ple. Within broad national guidelines, which the federal government provides, each of the states carries out the following activities:

- Establishes its own eligibility standards
- Determines the type, amount, duration, and scope of services to be covered
- Sets the rate of payment for services
- Administers its own program

## Program of All-Inclusive Care for the Elderly (PACE)

An optional benefit under both Medicare and Medicaid is the Program of All-Inclusive Care for the Elderly (PACE). PACE focuses entirely on older adults who are frail enough to meet their state's standards for nursing home care. It features comprehensive medical and social services that can be provided at an adult day health center, at home, and/or at inpatient facilities.

For most clients, the comprehensive service package permits the frail elderly person to continue living at home while receiving services rather than being institutionalized. A team of physicians, nurses, and other health professionals assesses the client's needs, develops care plans, and then delivers all services, which are integrated into a complete health care plan. PACE is available only in states that have chosen to offer PACE under Medicaid.

Eligible individuals who wish to participate enroll voluntarily. PACE enrollees must meet the following requirements:

- Be at least fifty-five years of age
- Live in the PACE service area
- Be screened by a team of primary-care physicians, nurses, and other health professionals, including dietitians; physical, occupational, and recreational therapists; social workers; and personal care attendants
- Sign and agree to the terms of the enrollment agreements

PACE offers and manages all of the medical, social, and rehabilitative services their enrollees need to preserve or restore their independence, to remain in their own homes and communities, and to maintain their quality of life. The PACE service package must include all Medicare and Medicaid services provided by that state. At a minimum, there are an additional sixteen services that a PACE organization must provide, including social work, drugs, and nursing facility care. Benefits include a broad range of therapies and assistance. When an enrollee is receiving adult day care services, meals and transportation are also covered. Aid is usually provided in an adult day health setting, but it may also include in-home and other needed referral services.

The PACE team has daily contact with enrollees. This helps team members detect subtle changes in enrollees' condition, so the team can respond quickly to medical, functional, and psychosocial problems.

PACE receives a fixed monthly payment per enrollee from Medicare and Medicaid. The amounts are the same during the contract year, regardless of the services an enrollee may need. Persons enrolled in PACE also may have to pay a monthly premium, depending on their eligibility for Medicare and Medicaid. Currently there are twenty-five PACE sites, and each site has about 100 enrollees. Limited new sites may be added each year.

> *The official Medicare website is www.medicare.gov. Many helpful documents are available through this site, including one on alternatives to nursing home care. The search function is very useful as well—simply type in what you are looking for, such as "alternatives to nursing homes."*

## Social Health Maintenance Organizations (S/HMOs)

A social HMO is an organization that provides the full range of Medicare benefits offered by standard HMOs plus additional services:

- Care coordination
- Prescription drugs
- Homemakers
- Personal care services
- Adult day care
- Medical transportation
- Respite care
- Chronic care (short-term nursing home care)

Other services (such as eyeglasses, hearing aids, and dental benefits) may also be provided. These plans offer the full range of medical benefits that are offered by standard HMOs plus chronic-care and extended-care services. Membership offers other health benefits that are not provided through Medicare alone or most other senior health plans.

At the present time, four S/HMOs are participating in Medicare, and each S/HMO has eligibility criteria. These plans are located in Portland, Oregon; Long Beach, California; Brooklyn, New York; and Las Vegas, Nevada. As mentioned previously, the website www.benefits checkup.org offers quick and confidential searches and eligibility screening for programs that range from health coverage to supplemental income.

## Long-Term Care Insurance

Long-term care insurance is a type of coverage under which an insurance company pays for long-term care. Policyholders pay premiums to the company, and if the policyholder needs long-term care, the insurance company pays according to the contract provisions. Many companies provide some form of long-term care insurance, and their contracts have different provisions.

Since people are living longer because of advanced medical technology, pharmaceutical developments, and healthier lifestyles, there will be more opportunity for chronic disorders to develop and potentially restrict independent living. Currently, more than 1.5 million adults reside in assisted-living facilities, and the 6 million older adults who live at home need regular assistance from family and other sources.

The Health Care Financing Administration, the federal agency that oversees Medicare and Medicaid, states that approximately one-third of all long-term care costs are privately paid. About 40 percent of expenses are covered by Medicaid, but only after the resident's assets have been depleted. Consumers view long-term care insurance as a means of protecting assets and avoiding dependency on family members for care in old age.

A consumer interested in this type of coverage should begin by contacting the state insurance commission and obtaining the state's booklet describing guidelines for long-term care insurance. The Eldercare Locator Service (800-677-1116) provides telephone numbers for state and local agencies in each state. Two other organizations provide additional resources: for a copy of "A Shopper's Guide to Long-Term Care Insurance" write to the National Association of Insurance Commissioners, 120 W. 12th Street, Suite 1100, Kansas City, MO 64105 and for "A Consumer's Guide to Long-Term Care Insurance," contact the Health Insurance Association of America, P.O. Box 41455, Washington, D.C. 20018.

# Alternatives to Nursing Home Care

Both PACE and S/HMOs offer useful options through Medicare to elders who are considering long-term care. Nursing homes serve as permanent residences for people who are too frail or sick to live at home or who need a temporary facility during a recovery period. Yet many people who need the nursing home level of care prefer to remain in their own home, assisted by family and friends, community services, and professional care agencies.

Medicare provides limited access to PACE and S/HMO coverage for designated beneficiaries needing comprehensive medical and social service delivery without residential placement.

Some people, however, require less than skilled care, or require skilled care for only short periods of time. Most communities have a variety of living arrangements that provide different levels of care. Before deciding on a care setting, older adults should talk with a physician or social worker about the level of care needed. While most people would choose to stay at home, it is important that all involved clearly understand the amount of responsibility and work required when that choice is made.

## Adapting an Older Adult's Home for Safety and Comfort

A long and healthy life is everyone's goal. Most persons in the United States today can look forward to spending a significant number of years in old age. Whether these years will be healthy, with high levels of physical and cognitive functioning, and the ability to live independently with access to affordable health care is of prime concern to elders and their families.

Most older adults would opt for independent living as opposed to residential placement. The Administration on Aging's fact sheet "Action Ideas for Older Persons and Their Families" details how, in selected situations, home modification and repair may allow people to remain safely in their own homes with increased comfort and lifestyle accommodations. Changes in home design can make it easier and safer to carry out activities of daily living such as bathing, cooking, and climbing stairs. Adaptation alone often can enable frail elders to remain at home.

More than 60 percent of older adults live in homes that are more than twenty years old. Moreover, the older homes these elders live in usually need to be repaired and modified. Appropriate alterations to meet the needs of the elderly residents can prevent one-third to one-half of home accidents, a significant risk factor in the life of frail elderly. Table 8.2 identifies modifications that can solve typical problems. Other easily implemented home adaptations that remove barriers to independent living and improve home safety are repositioning shelves, installing a full-length bathroom mirror, rearranging furniture, and removing high-pile, low-density carpeting.

### Table 8.2 Modifications to Create a Safer Home Environment

| Typical Problem | Possible Solution |
| --- | --- |
| Difficulty getting in and out of the shower | Install grab bars and transfer benches |
| Slipping in tub or shower | Place nonskid strips or decals in tub and shower |
| Awkward faucet handles, doorknobs | Replace knobs with lever handles |
| Inadequate heating, ventilation | Install insulation, storm windows, air conditioning |
| Difficult access to home | Install ramps |
| Problems climbing stairs | Install handrails for support |
| Difficulty sitting on toilet | Install grab bars and raised toilet seat |
| Need for wheelchair accommodation | Install offset hinges to widen doorways |

The older adult can undertake a home modification and repair plan in three ways: doing the project with a friend or relative, hiring a contractor, or contacting a home modification and repair program.

An older adult who chooses to hire a contractor should be careful to select a licensed and bonded contractor. The homeowner should secure bids from several contractors and examine references. If possible, the homeowner should inspect a project that the contractor has completed. Having a family lawyer or other reliable third party study a written contract helps to protect the elder from fraud. Other sources of reference regarding a contractor's reliability and performance record are the local Better Business Bureau and the city or county's consumer affairs office.

## Financial Assistance

Programs exist that offer loans or free services to eligible elderly individuals who wish to modify or repair their homes. For more information, contact the following agencies:

- *Farmers Home Administration*—The agency offers grants and loans to low-income rural elderly.
- *Community Development Department*—Many cities and towns use Community Development Block Grants to help citizens maintain and upgrade their homes.
- *Local welfare or energy departments*—Two programs, the Low-Income Home Energy Assistance Program (LIHEAP) and the Weatherization Assistance Program (WAP) of the U.S. Department of Energy, provide funds to weatherize the homes of lower-income persons.
- *Health care providers*—Funds from Medicare and Medicaid are available for a wide array of durable medical equipment with a physician's prescription.
- *Local Area Agency on Aging*—Funds from the Older Americans Act, Title III, often can be used to modify and repair homes.
- *Local banks and lenders*—Some banks and lenders offer home equity conversion mortgages, which allow homeowners

to turn the value of their homes into cash without having to move or to make regular loan payments.

## Reverse Mortgages

A *reverse mortgage* is a type of home loan that allows homeowners to convert the equity in their home into cash. This option affords older adults greater financial security by providing the cash to supplement Social Security, manage unexpected medical expenses, and underwrite home improvements.

Homeowners who are sixty-two and older and who have paid off their mortgages, or who have only small mortgage balances remaining, are eligible to participate in the U.S. Department of Housing and Urban Development's (HUD's) reverse mortgage program. Applicants can elect to receive payments in a lump sum, on a monthly basis (for a fixed term or for as long as they live in the home), or on an occasional basis such as a line of credit. If the homeowners' circumstances change, they can restructure the payment options.

Unlike ordinary home equity loans, a HUD reverse mortgage does not require repayment, as long as the borrower lives in the home. Lenders recover their principal plus interest when the home is sold. The remaining value of the home goes to the homeowner or to his or her survivors. If the proceeds of the sale do not cover the amount owed, HUD makes up the shortfall. An insurance premium collected from all borrowers by the Federal Housing Administration (part of HUD) provides this coverage.

The FHA's reverse mortgage insurance makes HUD's program less expensive to borrowers than the smaller reverse mortgage programs run by private lenders without FHA insurance.

*Beware of fraudulent lenders that charge thousands of dollars for information that is free from HUD. To report fraud or abuse in the reverse mortgage program, call toll-free 1-888-466-3487.*

## *Renters*

Renters are not excluded from assistance. The Fair Housing Act of 1988, Section 6(a), makes it illegal for landlords to refuse to let tenants make reasonable modifications to their house or apartment if the tenant is willing to pay for the remodeling. For more information, check state government websites for specific housing regulations or contact an eldercare resource service, such as Eldercare Locator.

# Special Considerations for Elderly Minorities

Upcoming shifts in the racial/Hispanic composition of the elderly population will necessitate special consideration when preparing for long-term care. As noted in earlier chapters, ethnic minorities will be a growing share of the U.S. elderly population. The rapid growth of minority groups will heighten the need for special services accommodating their characteristic cultural features in several areas:

- Knowledge of English
- Living arrangements
- Income
- Education

Federal and state governments and long-term care facilities are only partially prepared to meet the needs of minorities. The increase in the minority population demands more timely preparation. For example, elderly Native Americans (including American Indians, Eskimos, and Aleuts) reside in each of the fifty states and the District of Columbia. They are 8 percent of the total 2 million American Indians. Because of their small numbers and wide geographic distribution, alerting this special group of the elderly to services consists of targeting Older Americans Act programs, creating ways for state and area Agencies on Aging to inform widely scattered groups of people about local programs and services, and ensuring that the programs administered under Title III are available to all eligible recipients.

Outreach to underserved communities is more effective when it includes respecting and acknowledging traditions and beliefs. For example, elderly Hispanics and Native Americans characteristically have been cared for by their families and tend to "trust in faith" that everything will work out. For them, the necessary services may require a different structure and orientation reflecting these ethnic conventions.

# Making the Long-Term Care Decision

The need for long-term care is based on the limitations of a person's ability to manage certain functions. For example, a client with a chronic condition might require assistance with activities of daily living such as bathing, dressing, and toileting. The type of assistance might be one-on-one assistance or supervision and cueing from another person. Other clients have restrictions that are inconvenient but not as limiting. Difficulties in managing money, cleaning, grocery shopping, and taking medication are referred to as limitations in instrumental activities of daily living.

Individuals with impairments in either category vary widely in severity and frequency. An estimated 2 million elderly persons live in the community with severe physical and cognitive disabilities for which they need help and supervision. Another 1.6 million live in nursing homes. While only 5 percent of the elderly population reside in nursing homes, as people age, the likelihood they will need this type of care increases. It is estimated that half of the U.S. population will require some type of long-term care during their lives. This includes nursing home, assisted living, home health care, and rehabilitation facility care.

# The Caregiver Picture

Women, usually daughters, tend to provide most of the informal care of the impaired older adult. Secondary caregivers are few in number and provide much less care. When they do help, it is on an intermittent basis. The secondary caregivers are most often the spouse or children of the primary caregiver. This concentration of responsibilities on a nuclear family has obvious implications for problems within the family, which, in turn, increase the risk for the institutionalization of the impaired elderly person. The following examples illustrate the range of challenges, as well as some coping strategies.

Kate, fifty, had to move her elderly mother, Hannah, into an assisted-living setting. Hannah could no longer drive, often forgot meals, and was unable to adhere to a medication schedule. Kate thought that the charming residence and the willing employees were an answer to her prayers. At first, Hannah seemed enthusiastic. She liked the idea of being close to her only child, and she anticipated seeing more of her two grandchildren. Kate breathed a sigh of relief; her mother was close—no longer 600 miles away—and someone was making sure she had her meals and her medicine on time.

Kate hadn't counted on being called at home and at work ten to fifteen times a day and listening to rambling, repetitive conversations. Even though she visited several times a week, her mother claimed she was lonely because she didn't know anyone and never had any visitors. She complained that she should never have left her lovely old Victorian home in the Midwest. Although she admitted the residence was lovely and the workers there were very gracious, she said she had changed her mind and wanted to go home.

Kate experienced guilt, stress, and resentment at being interrupted with the same litany of regrets daily. Although her mother lives in a residential setting, Kate knows firsthand the stresses that afflict the "sandwich generation." The pressures of managing her own family obligations and the irritation at her mother for the relentless repetition of complaints often interfere with Kate's work responsibilities.

Kate probably can't change her mother's behavior, but she can alter her own. She might begin by screening her calls at work. And she should get a large calendar, hang it in a prominent place in her mother's residence, and note the days she visits or will visit on the calendar to jog her mother's memory. Support groups and chat rooms are available for exchanging tips on managing the problems and frustrations caused by having a loved one with dementia.

Liz, an unmarried forty-eight-year-old schoolteacher, has always lived at home with her widowed mother. When seventy-eight-year-old Margaret fell and broke her hip, Liz's family and friends urged her to seek residential placement, citing her mother's projected needs and Liz's job requirements. Liz, a resourceful, energetic only child, wouldn't hear of it.

The mother was discharged from the hospital and had rehabilitative services at home. In time, she managed to get around quite well in a wheelchair. She retained some ambulatory skills but remained at high risk for falls. In fact, she fell several times while transferring herself from wheelchair to toilet, sustaining multiple bruises but, fortunately, no additional fractures. Margaret was also hospitalized periodically for dehydration, urinary tract infections, and "spells" in which she spoke incoherently and didn't recognize her daughter. Nevertheless, she remains alone at home with a portable phone in her lap, refusing all outside help except for a weekly cleaning woman. She has bouts of depression yet is immeasurably buoyed by her daughter's devoted and unflagging attention and frequent visits from friends.

Margaret could improve this situation by scheduling visits from a home health aide during the week. Margaret would enjoy the presence of a compatible person for an hour or two a day, and the hazards to her safety would be considerably reduced.

Gus, eighty-eight, lives with his wife, Lydia, eighty-two, in a small apartment in a midsized city. Lydia had a stroke that left her paralyzed on one side. Gus takes care of her with some help from a home health aide. He learned how to get Lydia in and out of bed and how to dress and toilet her. Meals-on-wheels dinners are delivered daily, but Gus is still able to shop and do simple cooking.

Gus's health also is impaired. He takes medications for both arthritis and hypertension. Some days when his arthritis is troubling him and his energy level is low, his disposition isn't as cheerful as it used to be. His two sons, who live in neighboring states, phone frequently and visit when they can. They see clearly that their father is increasingly frail and fatigued. Nevertheless, Gus is determined to keep Lydia with him as long as possible and credits this decision with her recovery and ability to manage simple functions.

Gus may consider increasing the hours of the home health aide. Lydia is also a candidate for a temporary respite setting, and that would give Gus a well-deserved rest.

Of the three caregivers, the one bearing the heaviest brunt of caregiver strain and exhibiting the effects of his burden is Gus. According to a 1999 study reported in the *Journal of the American Medical Association* by Richard Schultz and Scott Beach, the physical demands of caregiving and the frailties of elderly caregivers heighten the risk for poor health and a greater mortality. They conclude that being a caregiver who endures mental and emotional stress because of the caregiving responsibilities contributes to increased depression. Prolonged distress coupled with the demands of caregiving expand the physical vulnerabilities of the frail elder committed to the mission of caregiving.

Family caregivers are an indispensable national resource, with approximately 15 million adults providing care to relatives. If the work of these caregivers had to be replaced by paid home care staff, the cost would be between $45 and $75 billion per year. In the case of Alzheimer's disease, the crippling form of dementia described in Chapter 6, it is estimated that more than half are being cared for in the community. Between 2.5 million and 3.1 million spouses, relatives, and friends are caregivers, and they form the basic structure of the nation's informal caregiving community.

As shown in Figure 8.1, family caregivers have always been the linchpin of long-term care for impaired elderly relatives or friends. For older adults living in the community who need some assistance with activities of daily living, fully 95 percent have some family members involved in their care. Despite marked changes in present-day family dynamics (for example, more women in the paid workforce and increased geographic separation), families manage innovatively to care for their older relatives.

The most recent National Long Term Care Survey, augmented by other research, indicates the following facts about the burden shouldered by these caregivers:

- Caregivers dedicate about twenty hours per week to providing care for older adults, a figure that increases when the older person has multiple impairments.
- Caregiving is physically stressful. It can involve heavy lifting and turning, frequent linen changes, increased laundry, and

**Figure 8.1  Sources of Assistance for Impaired Elders**

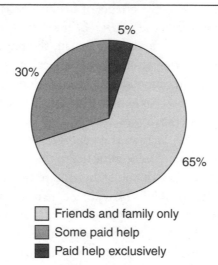

| | Friends and family only |
| | Some paid help |
| | Paid help exclusively |

toileting the elder. These activities often deplete the physical reserves of the caregiver, who may also be elderly.

- Assuming the long-term care responsibilities for impaired elderly relatives or friends can impose emotional strain on the caregiver. Such strain often results in depression.

- Two-thirds of working caregivers state that work schedules and caregiving often conflict. The resulting disruptions often compel them to work fewer hours and/or take unpaid leaves of absence.

## Caregiver Support

In recognition of the indispensable contribution of families, and to aid families in their caregiving efforts, the federal budget for fiscal year 2000 proposed a National Family Caregiver Support Program as one of four long-term care initiatives. Under this proposed Older Americans Act program, the state Offices (or Units or Departments) on Aging, together with local Area Agencies on Aging, community service providers, and consumer organizations, will be expected to put into place five program components:

1. Provision of information to caregivers about available services
2. Assistance to caregivers in gaining access to such services
3. Individual counseling, organization of support groups, and provision of caregiver training to help families make decisions and solve problems relating to their caregiver roles
4. Respite care to give families and other informal caregivers temporary relief from their caregiving responsibilities
5. Supplemental long-term care services, on a limited basis, to complement the care provided by family caregivers and other informal caregivers

One of the first resources a caregiver should consult when needing help is the local Area Agency on Aging. These agencies are listed in the city or county government sections of the telephone directory under "aging" or "social services." Their function is to serve the local community, the elderly residents, and their families.

The value of caregiver support programs cannot be underestimated. Their goal is to diminish the stress associated with the protracted demands of caring for an older person. Participating in a caregiver support program gives caregivers access to information and maintains or improves their morale.

## Ethnic Groups and Caregiving

In the last ten years, there has been increasing attention to differences in caregiving across ethnic groups. Early studies focused mainly on comparisons of African-Americans and whites. More recently, researchers have also studied Hispanic and Asian-American subgroups.

The incidence of caregiving is higher among minorities. The studies suggest that the larger and modified extended families of African-Americans and Hispanics increases the informal care resources of elderly persons in these two groups. Furthermore, caregivers in these three minority groups are more likely than in the general population to provide care for more than one person. As detailed in Table 8.3, they are also more apt to be living with the person they care for and to have help from other persons.

**Table 8.3 Living Arrangements of the Population Aged 65 and Older, by Sex and Race and Hispanic Origin, 1998**

| | With Spouse | With Other Relatives | With Non-Relatives | Alone |
|---|---|---|---|---|
| **Men** | | | | |
| Total | 72.6 | 7.0 | 3.0 | 17.3 |
| White | 74.3 | 6.0 | 2.7 | 17.0 |
| Black | 53.5 | 14.8 | 6.8 | 24.9 |
| Asian and Pacific Islander | 72.0 | 20.8 | 0.6 | 6.6 |
| Hispanic | 66.8 | 15.0 | 4.3 | 14.0 |
| **Women** | | | | |
| Total | 40.7 | 16.8 | 1.7 | 40.8 |
| White | 42.4 | 14.8 | 1.6 | 41.3 |
| Black | 24.3 | 32.2 | 2.7 | 40.8 |
| Asian and Pacific Islander | 41.3 | 36.7 | 0.8 | 21.2 |
| Hispanic | 36.9 | 33.8 | 1.8 | 27.4 |

Note: These data refer to the civilian noninstitutional population. Hispanics may be of any race.

Source: Census Bureau, *Current Population Survey*, March 1998.

## Caregiving and the Employer/Employee Relationship

In 1999 the National Council on Aging conducted a survey of 1,300 employees of a large company, using an anonymous, voluntary questionnaire. The average age of the respondents was forty-one; approximately two-thirds were women. Among respondents, 80 percent of caregivers who lived with an older adult spoke daily to that person, compared to 17 percent of those who lived 100 miles or more from the care recipient. Many caregivers from each group reported that the elderly relative for whom they were responsible would call several times a day, disrupting their work.

Caregivers were asked to indicate the services they viewed as essential to them over a twelve-month period. As shown in Table 8.4, the most widely valued services were those related to information about locating or monitoring various programs and benefits. Other important services were transportation, shopping, and household chores.

### Table 8.4 Types of Assistance Caregivers Request

| Services Needed | Percentage of Caregivers Who Request/Need the Service |
|---|---|
| Locating various programs and benefits | 69% |
| Monitoring programs and benefits | 64% |
| Transportation arrangements | 60% |
| Shopping | 58% |
| Household chores | 54% |
| Outside home maintenance | 53% |
| Medical insurance forms and reimbursments | 51% |
| Finding legal information | 49% |
| Arranging relief from caregiving | 49% |
| Meal preparation | 44% |
| Locating assessment specialists for medical and emotional needs | 44% |
| Locating safe, supervised adult daycare | 40% |
| Day-to-day financial coordination | 38% |
| Bathing | 35% |

## Types of Assistance Caregivers Value

The survey also asked employee caregivers to propose services or actions by employers that would assist them in their caregiver roles. The employees provided the suggestions listed in Table 8.5.

### Table 8.5 Help Employee Caregivers Want from Their Employers

- A stated corporate policy for caregivers
- Flexibility in scheduling
- Help in planning for elder care, especially as needs increase
- A single phone number to call to initiate a search for resources
- Checklist and guides to help families manage crisis situations and caregiving in general
- Translation of industry jargon into plain English
- Reliable, objective means of evaluating different caregiver services
- More affordable services, more user-friendly billing

# The Nursing Home Setting

Serious health impairments often lead to nursing home admission because of the complexity of the problems families encounter when trying to manage the care of an individual at home. Included in the severely disabled category are individuals with clinically diagnosed Alzheimer's disease. In time, most Alzheimer's patients wander, get lost, have altered sleep patterns, become incontinent, and engage in other behaviors that indicate a need for intense support. These behaviors drain families' physical and emotional resources.

This decision to seek nursing home placement is made when caregivers reach the limits of social, financial, and housing resources. Furthermore, nursing home placement, like the progression of Alzheimer's disease, increases with advancing years. The concentration of women in nursing homes is very high. With the proportion of women in each age group growing as age increases, that pattern will most likely continue.

The nursing home industry is a key element in the long-term care continuum providing residential care for the elderly. For many older adults needing intermediate levels of care, long-term care is provided in the home by relatives and friends and in small-group settings. However, nursing homes will continue to be used by those who need sophisticated labor-intensive twenty-four-hour skilled supervision. As a result, the potential market for this service will continue to be substantial.

In 1997 the Centers for Disease Control and Prevention and the National Center for Health Statistics published data from the 1995 National Nursing Home Survey. According to the study, about 1.5 million residents were being cared for in nearly 17,000 nursing homes. More than 35 percent of the residents were over eighty-five. The residents were also predominantly white (88 percent) and female (72.3 percent).

The survey indicated that two-thirds of nursing homes are operated for profit. The large number of proprietary homes, which have the majority of nursing home beds, leads the nursing home segment of the health care delivery system.

Another important characteristic of a nursing home is its certification status. Homes may be certified by Medicare, Medicaid, or both. More than two-thirds of the nursing homes certified hold dual certification.

One of the most significant findings of this survey was the fact that it showed a decrease in the ratio of nursing home residents to elders in the general population. The prodigious growth of the home care industry, as an effort to control health care costs, demonstrates that many elderly are not going to nursing homes for care that they can receive and *prefer* to receive at home. Another explanation is that older adults were healthier in 1995 than older adults twenty years earlier.

# Choosing the Residence

The selection of appropriate residential placement for an older adult requires careful evaluation of several factors:

- Location
- Availability
- Staffing
- Medicare/Medicaid
- Services and fees
- Religious/cultural preferences
- Language
- Special care needs

## *Location*

If there are several nursing homes to evaluate, all other things being equal, select a residence that will be close to family and friends. Frequent visits relieve loneliness and can ease the transition to the nursing home for both the client and the family. Convenience makes it easier for elderly friends to keep in touch and acts as a time-saver for busy, pressured families. Equally important, visitors assume a necessary role as advocates for residents.

## Availability

Nursing homes have a limited number of beds. When an admission decision is made, the question then becomes, Does the client add his or her name to a waiting list, or is there immediate bed availability? While nursing homes do not have to accept all applicants for admission, they do have to comply with Civil Rights provisions that prohibit discrimination based on race, religion, sex, age, etc.

## Staffing

The people who work in nursing homes are caring for a vulnerable population. Licensed, professional staff must hold current licenses without any disciplinary action pending. This information is public and available through a state's Division of Registration. Ancillary staff needs to be properly trained, and all staff should have criminal background checks. (This is desirable, but not yet required.) Frail, elderly people are under their protective supervision. Inquire about the nurse/patient ratio and the nursing assistant/patient ratio.

## Paying for Care

Nursing home care is costly. For most people, trying to find a way to finance a family member's nursing home expenses is a serious concern. About half of all nursing home residents pay costs out of their savings. When their resources become depleted, the resident is then usually eligible for Medicaid. Some managed-care plans or employee health benefits cover nursing home expenses either fully or partially.

Determine whether the chosen nursing home accepts Medicare or Medicaid payment. Often a facility will save only a few beds for Medicare or Medicaid residents. Such designations are critical for private-paying clients. If a private-pay client changes to Medicaid during the course of his or her residence and Medicaid beds are not available, the resident is apt to be transferred to another facility.

## Services and Fees

Nursing homes are required to inform prospective residents in writing about services, charges, and fees before admission. Most facilities charge a basic rate that includes room, meals, basic nursing care, house-keeping, laundry, recreation activities, and some personal care services. Some commonly accepted extra charges are hairdresser/barber services and telephone installation, but there may be additional fees.

## Religious and Cultural Preferences

Long-term care choices may be influenced by religious practices and cultural traditions. Such qualifications, particularly dietary practices, are important considerations when selecting residences.

## Language

Residents should be able to communicate with the staff in their primary language. Inability to do so increases fear, loneliness, and depression.

## Special Care Needs

Nursing homes provide basic nursing care, yet applicants may have special medical needs or preferences. Physical, occupational, and speech therapies are usually available. Secured Alzheimer's units, ventilators, and primary mental illness diagnoses may not be available.

An individual's requirements and preferences also vary widely: for example, not all nursing homes offer pool therapy, and not all nursing homes are equipped to accept emergency admissions.

*Family members who visit nursing homes should request a copy of the most recent state inspection of the home. This report is a thumbnail sketch of the residence's compliance with federal safety and health regulations. Inspections take place approximately every nine to fifteen months.*

## Quality of Care

Nursing homes are legally mandated to assess each new resident thoroughly within two weeks of admission. This assessment includes documenting the newly admitted resident's physical and mental status, mobility limits, skin condition, nutritional state, and rehabilitation needs.

When the assessment is completed, the nursing home is then required to develop a resident care plan that helps each resident reach or maintain his or her highest level of well-being. Representatives of various disciplines within the facility plus the resident and the family participate in the care plan's completion. Care plans are dynamic and change as the resident's needs change.

## Quality of Life

Quality of life largely involves issues of control and freedom. Admission to a nursing home means that residents have conceded to themselves and their families that they can no longer care for themselves and are dependent on others for many basic needs. This relinquishing of control over one's daily life is traumatic and often resented.

A good nursing home setting recognizes an individual's need for some control over the events in daily life and makes every effort to involve residents in basic decisions whenever possible. For example, a resident should be allowed to choose whether to shower in the morning or in the evening. One man may like to go to bed at 7:30 P.M., but another may want to watch the 11:00 P.M. news. Whenever possible, individual differences should be respected.

## Questions Families Should Ask

Besides these basic issues, families should consider other questions that will help them ensure the elderly resident's well-being will be maintained. The following questions address some of these miscellaneous issues:

- If a resident shares a room, how is a roommate chosen? How are differences between roommates resolved?
- How are a resident's property and personal items protected?
- Are there a variety of activities for residents? Do they include nonambulatory persons?

- What is the policy for family members who want to bring in favorite foods for residents?
- Are there written policies to prevent resident abuse and neglect?

# After Admission

Adjusting to nursing home admission is usually difficult for new residents. Circumstances of admission, states of physical and mental health, and preparation (or lack of the same) influence this sensitive period of adjustment. The support of family and friends can ease the transition, as in the following example.

Annette, a frail eighty-two-year-old, had to move from a nursing home in her home city where she lived for thirty years to a different nursing home seventy-five miles away. She had only one son, and he wanted her to be closer to him and his family. She saw the wisdom of the decision at the time, but when the time came to move, she felt uneasy and afraid. It was hard trying to learn so many new names— again! Annette had another roommate to get used to and more landmarks to remember when she propelled herself in her wheelchair out to the dining room. Her son hung her pictures and brought her treasured easy chair and floor lamp to her room. Gradually, her surroundings began to look familiar. Her son and her daughter-in-law visited often, both together and separately, and Annette found the visits to be comforting. Nevertheless, she reminded her son that she *still* missed her former residence.

After a loved one has been admitted to a nursing home, families should visit the nursing home frequently and at different times. Some visits should be made in the evening and on weekends, because staffing patterns and caregiving are often different at these times.

## *Admissions Contracts:*
## *Rights of Patients and Their Families*

Some residents outlive their family, and remaining friends may be too frail to help with legal or financial matters. Nursing homes must provide *each* resident not only with assistance in contacting legal and financial professionals, but also with any needed counseling.

All residents are informed of important information regarding their rights in a nursing home admission contract. In brief, nursing homes are obliged to ensure residents' safety and to take responsibility for residents' loss of personal property. These contracts also state that residents have the right to refuse any treatment they do not want, but usually the resident must agree to routine day-to-day care involving such matters as personal hygiene and allowing rooms to be cleaned.

Patients in hospitals and residents of any long-term care facility are supplied with a Patients' Bill of Rights. These rights include but are not limited to the following:

- The right to respectful and courteous treatment
- The right to receive understandable explanations of treatments and their alternatives
- The right to refuse treatment, medications, or dietary restrictions
- The right to privacy and confidentiality
- The right to form and participate in resident councils

Relatives of residents also have rights. Family members and legal guardians have the right to privacy when visiting the resident. They also have the right to meet with families of other residents and to join or address family councils.

Family members are allowed to participate in the development of their relative's care plan *if* the resident approves. Relatives who have legal guardianship of a nursing home resident have the right to examine all medical records concerning their loved one, as well as the right to make important decisions on that person's behalf. Sometimes, as in the following example, family members can make a significant difference in the quality of care provided.

Naomi, sixty-six, sustained permanent brain damage after a massive stroke. She spent weeks in the hospital, during which time her family approved a permanent tracheostomy to assist her breathing and a gastrostomy tube insertion so she could be fed a formula directly into the stomach. Naomi was transferred to a nursing home, where she received skilled nursing care.

At the time of Naomi's admission, the nursing home maintained a respiratory therapy department, and the care plan indicated that Naomi's breathing tube and dressing would be cared for by respiratory therapists. In time, the nursing home eliminated the respiratory therapy department as a cost-cutting measure. The nurses knew how to give Naomi her breathing treatments and manage her gastrostomy tube feedings. A therapist would remain on call as a consultant. This was much cheaper than supporting a whole department.

Naomi was not the only patient at the nursing home with this diagnosis and these required treatments. Families of other residents similarly affected met at the support programs sponsored by the nursing home, and they discussed their dismay at the new policy. They informed the nursing home administration that they were unanimously opposed to the decision to eliminate respiratory therapy, and they petitioned to have it restored. After negotiating with the families, the administration hired a respiratory therapist for each of the three shifts, thus ensuring twenty-four hours' coverage for all tracheostomy patients. The therapist would administer the breathing treatments, monitor all related equipment, and change the necessary dressings.

In summary, family and friends can make sure the resident receives good care. They do this by visiting often, getting to know the staff, expressing concerns to the right staff member, and becoming active in the nursing home's family council.

## Protection of the Rights of Older Adults

If the family does not address the concerns of a family member or of a resident, the situation may be managed by informing the state's inspection agency or the long-term care ombudsman. For nearly thirty years, state ombudsman programs have investigated complaints and protected the rights of residents in nursing homes and board-and-care facilities. Furthermore, they have alerted the public, policy makers, and regulatory agencies to many conditions that required change in order to improve the health, safety, rights, and welfare of the residents.

In 1996 ombudsmen opened more than 126,000 new cases. Of the cases closed, 81 percent involved nursing homes. The five most frequent nursing home complaints concerned the following problems:

- Improper handling of accidents
- Failure to heed requests for assistance
- Neglect of personal hygiene
- Lack of respect for residents; poor staff attitudes
- Lack of adequate care plan or resident assessment

Another 17 percent of the cases closed involved board-and-care homes, including assisted living, adult care, and similar levels of care facilities. Complaints involving these settings most often concerned the following issues:

- Dissatisfaction with the menu (quality, quantity, variation, choice of foods)
- Physical abuse
- Administration and organization of medications
- Lack of respect for residents; poor staff attitudes
- Equipment or building disrepair; poor lighting and safety hazards

Since the Older Americans Act was amended in 1975, every state has had a long-term care ombudsman program to investigate and resolve nursing home complaints. The program has also been working toward extension of services to board-and-care facilities and, in some areas, to those who receive professional care at home. Older adults who are residents of long-term care facilities, and the families of these residents, may contact an ombudsman through their State Unit on Aging or Area Agency on Aging to see if the long-term care ombudsman program in a given area can help in solving problems.

Not all residents in need of advocates have access to the attention and services of an ombudsman, however. In many parts of the United States, ombudsman visits to homes are erratic and infrequent, and there is little evidence of strategies to make the community aware of ombudsman services. Therefore, large numbers of long-term care residents do not know of the program and thus do not use it.

Ombudsmen generally provide timely responses to complaints. Nevertheless, there are major problems in some localities. For example, some states administer the program through toll-free telephone service. In these situations, ombudsmen investigate the complaints through telephone inquiries exclusively. This places long-term care residents at a disadvantage, because many are reluctant to discuss their health, safety, welfare, and rights over the phone, and many are too frail or cognitively impaired. To fulfill their mission, ombudsman programs must make their services available and accessible to all residents of long-term care nursing facilities and board-and-care facilities.

# The Future of Long-Term Care Services

Long-term care, the aggregation of services provided to elders with chronic health conditions, differs from other types of health care in that the goal is not the cure of the chronic illness. Rather, the goal is to allow the stricken individual to reach and maintain an optimal level of functioning. A second important distinction from traditional health care is that long-term care includes services that are social as well as medical. An appropriate mix of health and social services is the most effective way to meet alterations in an individual's needs.

Life expectancy will probably increase substantially, even at older ages. Furthermore, there will also most likely be large increases in the number of older adults with poor health and with disabilities, including dementias such as Alzheimer's disease. As a result, demands on nursing home care and home care will intensify, if only because of the projected population expansion.

Survivors at the most advanced ages are mostly widowed females, owing to the premature death of men and the low remarriage rates of elderly women. Compared to other segments of the elderly population, this group tends to have a lower income, greater poverty, poorer health, and greater risk of institutionalization.

These facts suggest some means of moderating the requirements and expense of supporting dependent elderly: substituting home care for nursing home care when practical; judiciously using families, friends, and neighbors as caregivers; and bringing about a reduced death rate of married men in midlife.

# 9

# End of Life and Bereavement

EVEN WITH GREATER life expectancies and the best of health care, the aging process does inevitably end with death. Dying and death present extraordinary challenges to the dying person and his or her loved ones.

The advances in technology and biomedical research have created a wide array of choices for care and treatment at the end of life. At the same time, decisions about the management of final illnesses have also become much more complicated.

Patients and their families should have open discussions so everyone is aware how much or how little is to be done to maintain or extend life. However, these discussions may not completely satisfy the perceived needs of dying patients and their families. Treatment choices aside, their primary concerns are satisfactory pain control and clear communication.

*If your doctor's training was typical, information on death and dying was integrated into other courses. Few doctors have taken a separate course in end-of-life care.*

The challenges of delivering appropriate care face all health care providers who are in contact with terminally ill older adults. The main specialty areas of medical practice that manage end-of-life care are internal medicine, family medicine, neurology, and anesthesia. Whatever the doctor's specialty, the strategies of care must be tailored to fit the needs of the patient. The end-of-life needs of a patient dying from colon cancer clearly are different from the needs of the Alzheimer's patient dying from stroke. Cardiovascular disease and cancer are the leading causes of death in the United States. Since so many Americans are living past the age of sixty-five, many elderly die of these illnesses complicated by dementia.

*Every American has the constitutional right to request that medical treatment be withheld or withdrawn.*

# Pain Management

Although the medical specialties have differing perspectives of patients' requirements, there is a consensus of understanding on some basic principles of end-of-life care. One of the first principles, acknowledged by all health care professionals, is the relief of pain and other physical symptoms. Providing this relief is called *palliative care*. Comfort care or palliative care is care that eases or relieves a patient's symptoms without correcting the underlying causes of disease. Charles von Gunten, M.D., Ph.D., medical director of the Center for Palliative Studies at the San Diego Hospice, states, "Palliative care is interdisciplinary care focused on relieving suffering and improving quality of life."

Palliative care includes not only pain management, but also bereavement support, planning, and decision making. Ideally, palliative care honors the decisions made by dying patients and encourages mutual support among patients, families, and the health care personnel involved in solving problems and making choices regarding treatment. Palliative care also supports the spiritual needs of family members by providing pastoral care for those who express an interest in such guidance. Many patients and family members find that speaking to a trained spiritual caregiver helps them develop inner resources for healing and well-being.

> *In 1997 the Institute of Medicine's Committee on Care at the End of Life recommended that palliative care should become, if not a medical specialty, at least an area of expertise, education, and research.*

Despite medical progress, unacceptable numbers of critically ill elderly still die in hospitals and in pain, along with other distressing symptoms. Even when death is the unavoidable conclusion of a patient's illness, appropriate comfort measures often are not fully implemented. Caring for the dying patient requires that health providers change their mission from conventional aggressive treatment to palliative care. This is a difficult transition for many to make. A 1999 report before the House Committee on Government Reform revealed that while the technical advances in health care steadily lengthened life expectancy, research and attention to the quality of life and the experience of dying lagged behind. Not only was pain undertreated, but an individual's preference for "do not resuscitate" often was not honored. Families told of disruption caused by transferring a loved one from the hospital to a nursing home after technology prolonged life.

In response, there is a trend taking place in which many families are delivering patient care at home. These families frequently need assistance with skills training, problem solving, and information about the community-based services to which they are entitled.

Symptoms of distress common among terminally ill patients are pain, anxiety, breathing difficulties, cognitive disturbances, and weight loss. Care that focuses on relief of these symptoms enhances well-being and maximizes the quality of life for the dying patient.

Such patients and their families need reassurance that many palliative interventions are available.

In addition to traditional medicine, behavioral approaches to pain management can increase comfort in selected situations. Some examples are guided imagery (in which, for example, cancer patients imagine that their immune cells are attacking the malignancy) and relaxation techniques. Researchers in various disciplines are devoting increasing attention to measuring the relief given to terminally ill patients by adding alternative therapies to conventional care. They are finding that patients can learn to distinguish between dyspnea (difficulty in breathing) caused by anxiety and dyspnea due to physical causes. Acupuncture, massage therapy, and nutritional supplements appear to benefit certain patients with chronic obstructive pulmonary disease and congestive heart failure in which labored breathing is a major problem. Not only does patients' comfort increase, but patients feel the reward of actively participating in the management of their disease.

The National Cancer Institute is currently conducting research concerning palliative, hospice, and end-of-life care for patients. The care being studied involves a combination of drugs and behavior therapy. The study is investigating patient and family communication, decision making, ethics and clinical decisions, and caregiver support.

The Institute's goals are to improve the quality of care and to reduce the distress for caregivers. The tormenting symptoms once thought to be inevitable in a final illness can be relieved. Furthermore, the patient's autonomy, dignity, and quality of life can be improved and expanded. As Dr. Patricia Grady told the House Committee on Government Reform in 1999, "Complementary and conventional therapies have the potential to provide important information and new therapeutic approaches for improving care and quality of life at the end of life."

## Choosing the Type of Care

Curative and occasionally aggressive treatment is usually inappropriate for the terminally ill. Even so, some terminally ill patients choose such treatment—as is their right. Patients may even change their thinking about heroic measures to preserve life, to the consternation of family members and health care providers.

Ralph, fifty-nine, is a prime example. He had struggled with amyotrophic lateral sclerosis (ALS), also called Lou Gehrig's disease, for five years. He knew there was no cure, only symptomatic treatment, and that his prognosis was poor. In the early stages of his illness, Ralph decided he would refuse to consent to tube feeding when he could no longer swallow and to the use of a ventilator when he could no longer breathe on his own. After lengthy discussions with his family, his doctor, and his spiritual advisor, Ralph completed his advance directive to reflect these decisions. Yet, when the time came that he needed these invasive procedures in order to survive, Ralph insisted on having them done.

# Preparing for Emergencies

Emergency medical services (EMS), staffed by personnel referred to as emergency medical technicians (EMTs), are required to provide emergency care that prevents or limits complications from illness or injury prior to arrival at a receiving facility (hospital). However, rising numbers of people are choosing not to be resuscitated in the circumstances of cardiac or respiratory arrest. A conflict arises where there are no standard documents to help EMS personnel to recognize "do not resuscitate" (DNR) orders outside of a hospital setting. Patients needing immediate care and treatment are either unconscious or not competent under the circumstances. Emergency personnel are obliged to perform full resuscitative measures when called to the aid of a patient unable to inform them of their medical decisions.

A comfort care verification protocol has been designed to remedy this situation. It provides a standardized mechanism for the verifying of a DNR order so that technicians can recognize the order out of the hospital. Anyone (including minors) with a current valid DNR order is eligible for an order verification form and/or bracelet. Known as a CC/DNR order verification, it will include information such as the following:

- Patient's name, date of birth, gender, address, and signature
- Name and signature of guardian or health care agent
- Signature of physician or designee
- Issue and expiration dates

*Wearing a comfort care bracelet may also help protect very old, but not terminally ill persons, if they do not want CPR if they experience a cardiac or respiratory arrest. The placement of automated external defibrillators (AEDs) in public places gives the very old equal opportunity for having their hearts jump-started.*

Only physicians can request and receive CC/DNR forms from the department of public health, but they may give the forms to an authorized designee. EMS personnel will honor a current, valid CC/DNR order verification form or bracelet. They will provide noninvasive, full palliative care and transport the patient to a medical facility if appropriate.

## Advance Directives and Guardianship

Terminally ill patients should complete advance directives such as living wills, health care proxy, and durable power of attorney agreements. These documents provide instructions that relieve concerns about the kind of end-of-life care they prefer. The documents can ensure that if the individuals become incapacitated, their stated medical decisions will be honored.

Not only should individuals put their wishes in writing, they also should combine a living will and a durable health care power of attorney into a single document. Doing so helps the health care team, family, and friends to carry out the patient's wishes. The following examples illustrate topics that are often included in an advance directive:

- Cardiopulmonary resuscitation (CPR)—treatment done to restore breathing and heartbeat (may consist of vigorous chest compressions, electric shock to the chest, and the insertion of a breathing tube into the throat)
- Dialysis—a treatment used to cleanse the blood mechanically when kidneys do not function
- Ventilation—mechanical breathing treatment, using apparatus that provides respiration for patients unable to breath independently
- Artificial administration of food, water, or medications through tubes placed in the patient
- Organ donation

A sample advance directive appears at the end of this chapter.

## Advance Directives Defined

- *Living will*—indicates to family and physician which treatments you do not wish to have when you are near death
- *Health care proxy* (durable health care power of attorney)—names the person entrusted with your medical decisions when you are incapacitated
- *DNR*—"do not resuscitate" order

Although some individuals choose not to complete advance directives, any hospital or nursing home that receives Medicare or Medicaid funding must inform residents of their right to accept or to refuse treatment. In situations where there is no advance directive and the patient is incompetent due to dementia, the effects of critical illness, or the absence of relatives to contact, members of the medical staff become decision makers.

Respecting the rights of patients to refuse treatment and ensuring that they understand appropriate application of advance directives are important responsibilities of health care professionals.

The very old frequently need assistance managing their financial affairs because of the slow progression of cognitive deficits. If the behavior of an elder seems to be what others term "eccentric," that elder is vulnerable to the legal challenges of unscrupulous persons. If incompetence is demonstrated to a judge's satisfaction, the court appoints a guardian to supervise the elder's welfare.

A geriatric client's legal rights often are threatened in medical settings. If a very elderly patient rejects treatment deemed suitable by physicians, that decision raises conflicting questions about what is in the patient's best interests. Preparation of an advance directive makes physicians and their geriatric clients aware of options and preferences before the effects of drugs and illness cloud decision-making capabilities.

# Hospice

End-of-life care often involves a decision about hospice care. Conventional medical treatment focuses on curing illness through the use of medication, technology, and when indicated, surgery. The goals of hospice, in contrast, are pain control, comfort measures, and support of both patient and family. Most hospice care is provided in a patient's home, but the choice is also available in nursing homes and hospitals.

*About one-half of all Americans will spend some time in a long-term care facility. Many who require palliative care will live there in the final weeks and months of their lives.*

The expected outcome of hospice care is a comfortable, dignified death, not a return to health. All strategies aimed at achieving this goal are grounded in the appropriate management of the dying process of the patient and emotionally supportive aftercare for families. A hospice setting, whether at home, in a hospital, or in long-term care, also emphasizes more extensive personal attention and spiritual counseling given to patients before death and to families for one year after death.

A specifically prepared interdisciplinary team meets the medical, spiritual, and psychosocial needs of the dying patient. Provision is made for traditional services such as nursing care and the administration of medications needed to control pain. However, there are added benefits: social services, homemaker assistance, and in many cases, alternative healing skills such as acupuncture and massage therapy. Hospice agencies routinely provide the following services and equipment:

- Physician services and nursing care (on call twenty-four hours a day, seven days a week)
- Physical, speech, and occupational therapy
- Medical social worker services
- Medical supplies, such as dressings and catheters
- Drugs for symptom control and pain relief
- Equipment, including wheelchairs, commodes, and walkers
- Short-term care in a hospital or nursing home, including respite care and procedures necessary for pain control and symptom management
- Home health aide and homemaker services in some states
- Continuous home care of eight hours or more per day during a period of crisis as needed so that patients can remain in their homes (varies with different hospice organizations)
- Dietary counseling
- Counseling to help the hospice patient and family with grief and loss
- Any other item or service covered by Medicare

Hospice caregivers have contributed to the considerable reduction of some of the psychological distress experienced by bereaved family members. Family members have said the caregivers were always available, nonjudgmental, and clinically competent. Furthermore, they said communication between the professional caregiver and the family was effective. Psychological distress is a universal experience of bereavement. Yet giving the appropriate care prevented or at least reduced intense levels of this emotion.

## Pain Management in Hospice Care

Pain relief is the first priority for both patient and caregiver. Narcotics are used in most situations, and families have concerns about their use, because many people equate narcotics with "dope." They are repelled by the highly publicized stigma associated with the use of controlled drugs. Hospice reassures clients and encourages open communication among patients, families, and clinicians to improve patient care and decrease distress for caregivers.

Frequently questions concern the subjects of addiction, sedation, route of administration, and scheduling of administration:

- *Addiction*—Hospice patients receiving narcotics such as morphine are not addicts. When the patient's pain is well controlled, there is no craving for more of the drug.
- *Sedation*—Initially the administration of a narcotic may cause drowsiness. However, in a short period of time, the body of the terminally ill patient develops a resistance to sedation. Few patients who are well controlled are excessively drowsy. However, if this should occur, the dosage is adjusted or the doctor can prescribe a different medication.
- *Route of administration*—There is a widespread fear that the only way to administer a narcotic, such as morphine, is by injection. In fact, oral administration can achieve satisfactory pain control. If the patient cannot swallow the medicine, transdermal patches worn on the skin are comfortable, non-invasive alternatives.
- *Scheduling of drug administration*—Research has shown that regularly scheduled administration of pain medication results in better pain control. Furthermore, there is no upper

limit to prescribing opiates. Dosages can be increased to meet the patient's needs.

Families need to be reassured that narcotics such as morphine are not restricted to the last stages of an illness. Many people are maintained on morphine for extended periods of time with little disruption in their daily functioning.

## Medicare's Hospice Benefit

Medicare and Medicaid programs cover most hospice services for the terminally ill. The first question families and patients have about hospice is, How is eligibility determined? This benefit is available to anyone enrolled in Medicare Part A. The next qualifying factor is that the patient's physician and the hospice director must certify that the applicant is terminally ill with about six months or less to live. Patients who go into remission and leave hospice for a period of time can be readmitted at a later date. Of course, the ability to predict the duration of a terminal illness is limited. Therefore, patients who improve to the point where they no longer need the services of hospice are allowed to withdraw from the setting and to re-enroll for palliative care at a later date. Physicians recertify the patients every sixty days following the first two ninety-day periods of enrollment.

Medicare insures over 38 million Americans and nearly 90 percent of this population is sixty-five years of age or older. Not only is hospice a different kind of benefit than most enrollees exercise, but it is not widely used, despite enrollees' qualifications. Persons using hospice are generally older than the average Medicare population. The majority is made up of white males, and the predominant terminal illness is cancer.

One of the reasons hospice care is underutilized may be that health care providers have difficulty adjusting their professional philosophy from the usual goal of medicine (that of restoring the patient to health) to the hospice objective of focusing on the dying process. Physicians discuss the patient's preference to waive treatment and then certify that death is expected within six months. The hospice patient acknowledges life's endpoint and accepts comfort as the goal.

*Since November 1995, federal law requires hospitals and nursing homes to discuss hospice benefits at the time a patient is discharged.*

Using the Medicare hospice benefit in nursing homes improves the quality of care for the patients dying in these settings. The likelihood of adequate pain management is greater, fewer hospice patients are submitted to invasive treatments, and fewer hospice patients are hospitalized.

Most hospice patients are cared for at home. Some hospice patients choose to spend time in a hospice facility in order to give the caregiver at home some rest. Medicare will cover five consecutive respite days.

With the ability to improve dying residents' quality of life demonstrated so clearly through research, why are Medicare hospice benefits not more widely used? The research suggests that the predominant barriers are still the gaps in coordination between the hospice and the long-term care facility staff, as well as a lingering skeptical view of hospice care philosophies by some residents' physicians and the long-term care staff. Many nursing homes are building relationships with hospice programs, but stronger efforts need to be made to advance the initiative. The Medicare hospice benefit enables physicians and nursing home personnel to ensure the provision of comprehensive palliative care for terminally ill residents.

Together, patients and their families can maximize a palliative program decision by planning in advance for optimal end-of-life care.

# Funerals and Funeral Homes

No experience is more wrenching and disruptive than managing the after-death activities generated by the death of a loved one. The need to make most of the choices quickly adds to the stress and sorrow of the bereaved survivor. The family must decide whom to inform about the death, what type of service to select, where the deceased should be buried (or whether to bypass burial in favor of cremation). Each decision involves many emotional and legal questions.

The overriding concern of many families is the intimidating financial obligation. Whether the death is sudden or the result of a protracted illness, few individuals are ever really ready to pay for a funeral. Families spend billions of dollars annually in order to provide fitting funerals for their loved ones. This costly investment has prompted a steadily increasing trend toward preneed planning, that is, making funeral preparations in advance. Evidence indicates that consumers are taking steps to compare prices and services. The advantages are clear: the emotional expenditure is sharply reduced, since there is no decedent and the decision maker can give unhurried thought to personal preferences and to the future financial needs of survivors. In other words, the public is thoughtfully researching economic issues as well as creating suitable memorial tributes.

Common wisdom holds that the two most expensive purchases consumers make are homes and cars. Funerals rank a close third, since this tradition, including a casket and vault, costs on average about $6,000. Furthermore, that figure may not include the many extras:

- Cemetery site
- Opening of the grave
- Limousines
- Flowers
- Death certificates
- Obituary notices

This partial listing can add thousands of dollars to the survivors' financial liabilities.

Regardless of when an individual investigates funeral expenses—preneed or at the time of death—any comparison shopping is bound to be uncomfortable. It's especially difficult if grief clouds decisions about what constitutes showing the proper love and respect for the deceased.

## *Planning Ahead—or Not Planning*

Herbert, a seventy-three-year-old childless widower, collapsed in a local bank. After a few days in intensive care, he died. His only survivor was his niece Linda, the mother of two teenagers, who was left to make the funeral arrangements.

A funeral director escorted Linda and her husband into a room containing many styles of caskets, and they were overwhelmed by the variety. Looking at each other, they shrugged helplessly. "Well," said Linda, "Uncle Herbert always liked mahogany furniture, so I guess we should pick the mahogany casket." Mahogany caskets, like copper or bronze, can sell for as much as $10,000.

When eighty-six-year-old Benjamin passed away after a protracted illness, his eighty-eight-year-old wife was taken to the neighborhood funeral home by their surviving son. After they had selected a casket, the funeral director asked the widow what kind of clothing she would be bringing for the decedent. Benjamin had lost so much weight, she decided to buy a new suit. The son pointed out that a closed casket would save a considerable amount of money, as well as spare family and friends the shock of his altered appearance. Benjamin's wife insisted on the suit. "He was always so proud of the way he looked," she said. When the question of new shoes was raised, it was with great difficulty that the son persuaded his mother this was a totally unnecessary expense.

Like Benjamin's wife and Herbert's niece, many individuals spend indiscriminately in these situations assuming it is the proper way to demonstrate their feelings for the deceased. Advance planning is one way to eliminate hasty and unnecessary expenditures. For example, another important issue in planning any funeral is the disposition of remains. Given the short period of time between the death and the burial, distraught families often choose graves or cemetery plots without seeing what they are buying.

People determined to provide properly for their own families often see preplanning of funerals as another responsible action, somewhat related to estate planning and making a will. Taking such steps eliminates much of the stress endured by the bereaved family members, who otherwise would have to make these decisions under the heavy pressures of time and strong emotions. Preneed funeral plans can be made with a funeral home or through a funeral or memorial planning society. The latter is a nonprofit organization that provides information but not services.

Preplanning can be an emotional experience, even when there is no immediate need. It is difficult to view a display of coffins without relating it to one's personal mortality. Nevertheless, by comparing prices and services, consumers can make prudent yet respectful and satisfying decisions.

Persons considering prepayment for funeral goods and services should first get answers to the following questions, recommended by the Federal Trade Commission:

- What are you paying for? Are you buying merchandise only (such as a casket and a vault), or are you buying funeral services as well?
- What happens to the money you have prepaid? States have different requirements for handling funds paid for prearranged funeral services.
- What happens to the interest earned on money that is prepaid and put into a trust account?
- Are you protected if the firm you deal with goes out of business?
- Can you cancel the contract and get a full refund if you change your mind?
- What happens if you move to a different area or die while away from home? Some prepaid funeral plans can be transferred, but often at an added cost.

Regardless of what arrangement individuals make for their own funerals, it is clearly important that they inform their families. Otherwise, the decedent's wishes may not be fulfilled, or a bereaved survivor could end up paying for duplicate arrangements. Individual preferences should be written, and copies should be given to the family and to an attorney. Another copy should remain in a prominent place.

*Do not put funeral specifics in a will. Wills usually are not found or read until after the funeral. Do not put your wishes in a safe-deposit box, as the family may have to make arrangements on the weekend or a holiday, when the box cannot be opened.*

## *Choices*

Several factors determine the type of funeral a family chooses. The practices surrounding the way we care for our dead are based on cultural and religious traditions, as well as costs and personal preferences. After weighing these issues, the following questions can be answered satisfactorily:

- Will the funeral be elaborate or simple?
- Is a religious service indicated?
- Where and when will the service be held?
- Will there be a viewing?
- Will the remains be buried or cremated?

These are highly charged emotional decisions, usually made with the assistance of a funeral director. The majority of morticians are professionals who are truly interested in meeting their clients' needs, but some in the funeral provider business are guilty of inflating prices. To protect consumers, the Federal Trade Commission (FTC) imposes the Funeral Rule, which requires, among other regulations, that funeral directors give families itemized prices. This practice enables families to decide whether they want a "package" of commonly selected items or individual goods and services. The Funeral Rule has these additional requirements:

- You have the right to choose the funeral goods and services you want. (Some exceptions apply.)
- The funeral provider must state this right in writing on the general price list.

### Table 9.1 Planning for a Funeral

---

- *Shop around in advance.* Compare prices from at least two funeral homes. Remember that you can supply your own casket or urn.

- *Ask for a price list.* The law requires funeral homes to give you written price lists for products and services.

- *Resist pressure* to buy goods and services you don't really want or need.

- *Avoid emotional overspending.* It's not necessary to have the fanciest casket or the most elaborate funeral to properly honor a loved one.

- *Recognize your rights.* Laws regarding funerals and burials vary from state to state. It's a smart move to know which goods or services the law requires you to purchase and which are optional.

- *Apply the same smart shopping techniques you use for other major purchases.* You can cut costs by limiting the viewing to one day or one hour before the funeral, and by dressing your loved one in a favorite outfit instead of costly burial clothing.

- *Plan ahead.* It allows you to comparison shop without time constraints, creates an opportunity for family discussion, and lifts some of the burden from your family.

---

Source: from the Federal Trade Commission's booklet: *Funerals: A Consumer Guide*

- If state or local law requires you to buy any particular item, the funeral provider must disclose this fact on the price list, with a reference to the specific law.
- The funeral provider may not refuse, or charge a fee, to handle a casket you bought elsewhere.
- A funeral provider that offers cremations must make alternative containers available.

The FTC also has prepared the decision-making guidelines listed in the table. In addition, it operates an information number to handle complaints: 1-877-FTC-HELP (1-877 382-4357)

Three basic types of funeral services are offered to families: traditional, direct burial, and direct cremation. The traditional funeral is referred to as "full service." The director provides transportation, the casket, preparation of the body for viewing, and many incidentals that ease the emotional pressures on the bereaved. It is usually the most expensive type of funeral, because of the coordination of the many details involved. Direct burial typically includes the removal of the deceased from the place of death by the funeral home; care of the deceased until the day of burial; and transportation of the deceased to the cemetery the family selects. There is no viewing and no embalming. A funeral service may be held before or after the burial. Most families choose a simple graveside service or they may hold a memorial service at a future date. Direct cremation may be the simplest type of service. Cremation of the deceased proceeds without a viewing; memorial or other services are arranged by the family separately.

Long before Howard's last illness, Howard and Nancy had decided that they would choose to be cremated. They both felt that wakes, caskets, and all the floral tributes were unnecessary and personally distasteful. Yet when Howard died and Nancy attempted to make the arrangements, her adult children objected vigorously. They argued for a traditional funeral. Nancy consulted with the funeral director she and Howard had contracted with, and he suggested a compromise. Nancy agreed to a wake with an open casket. There would be a church service, but Howard would be cremated directly after the service. Nancy bypassed interment in a cemetery, choosing instead to scatter Howard's ashes at a future date in a favorite spot.

Later Nancy said, "I'm glad I was able to accommodate my children as well as myself. I didn't save any money with cremation, the way things turned out. Yet, looking back, this was the right decision for all of us."

Expenses related to purchasing cemetery plots mount quickly. The checklist details many possibilities. Grave liners, required in some areas, cost several hundred dollars. There are also costs to open and fill in graves. Families also must learn about regulations concerning monuments and maintenance. However, all veterans as well as their spouses and dependent children, are entitled to free burial and a grave marker in a national cemetery. For further information, contact the regional Veterans Administration office at 1-800-827-1000.

Most funeral providers are committed to meeting their clients' needs. Attentive listening and the willingness to be innovative and flexible increase the family's comfort and the provider's professional satisfaction.

### *Figure 9.1 Checklist for Shopping Funeral Homes*

---

**"Simple" disposition of the remains:**

_____   Immediate burial

_____   Immediate cremation

_____   If the cremation process is extra, how much is it?

_____   Donation of the body to a medical school or hospital

**"Traditional" full-service burial or cremation:**

_____   Basic services of the funeral director and staff

_____   Pickup of the body

_____   Embalming

_____   Other preparation of the body

_____   Least expensive casket

_____     Description, including model number

_____   Outer burial container (vault)

_____     Description

_____   Visitation/viewing—staff and facilities

_____   Funeral or memorial service—staff and facilities

_____   Graveside service, including staff and equipment

_____   Hearse

_____   Other vehicles

_____   Total

**Other services:**

_____   Forwarding the body to another funeral home

_____   Receiving the body from another funeral home

**Cemetery/mausoleum costs:**

_____   Cost of lot or crypt (if you don't already own one)

_____   Perpetual care

_____   Opening and closing the grave or crypt

_____   Grave liner, if required

_____   Marker/monument (including setup)

---

Source: from the Federal Trade Commission's booklet: *Funerals: A Consumer Guide.*

# Family Records

All families should keep certain important papers in fireproof, theft-proof storage. Examples of such documents are birth, marriage, and death certificates (several copies to identify a newly deceased spouse), tax returns, military records, leases, deeds, insurance policies, and copies of wills (originals should be on file in an attorney's office). Survivors have found that complete lists of all property—including real estate, stocks, bonds, savings accounts, and personal property of the deceased—are valuable systems to help in settling estates and to aid in the economic transition brought about by being widowed.

*Survivors should cancel credit cards that were in the deceased's name only. Also, contact the state department of motor vehicles to learn whether the title of a spouse's car needs to be changed.*

### Table 9.2 Resources for Common Family Documents

| | |
|---|---|
| Military personnel records (or lost military record) | National Personnel Records Center<br>Military Records Facility<br>9700 Page Avenue<br>St. Louis, MO 63132-5100<br>E-mail: center@stlouis.nara.gov |
| Pension benefits inquiry | Pension Benefits Guarantee Corporation<br>1200 K Street, N.W.<br>Washington, D.C. 20005-4026<br>1-800-827-1000 |
| Social Security retirement benefits | Local Social Security Administration office<br>1-800-772-1213 |
| Birth, death, marriage certificates | Local department of public health,<br>registry of vital records and statistics |

Note: For a complete checklist and personal inventory, see the end of this chapter.

Some documents, such as copies of insurance policies, are easy to replace, but others may be expensive and much more time-consuming to retrieve. Lack of access to such documents causes delays in the processing of benefits and adds needless stress to survivors and their families. Table 9.2 provides a starting point for obtaining important documents.

# Loss of a Spouse

The primary social relationship is that between spouses, and it is usually the strongest. When a spouse dies, the survivor's grief is likely to be intense. Feelings are physical and at times can be frightening. Surviving spouses have described digestive upsets, sleep disturbances, breathing difficulties, exhaustion, and other vague somatic complaints. Profound sadness often results in uncontrollable crying, at times when least expected.

The principal reactions to the loss of a spouse depend on several things: the quality of the relationship, psychological and spiritual resources, and the survivor's physical health. There are as many kinds of reactions as there are surviving spouses. However, some of the commonly shared emotions reported are disbelief, mental numbness, depression, guilt, and anger. Table 9.3 details common reactions to grief.

### Table 9.3  Common Elements of Grief

| Category | Example |
| --- | --- |
| Emotional | Sadness, frustration, shock, numbness |
| Physical | Fatigue, lack of appetite, insomnia |
| Behavioral | Social withdrawal, crying |
| Cognitive | Hallucinations, preoccupation |

Whether the death is sudden and unexpected or inevitable, as in the case of a long illness, the finality of the event always comes as a shock. The survivor's consciousness almost shuts down, and many of the necessary, immediate decisions are made automatically in a hazy, numbed state. There may be guilt if the bereaved person has regrets about the relationship or second-guesses the medical management of the deceased. Anger at being left alone is another normal reaction. Envy often accompanies anger—envy of those who still have their spouses.

The hours and days immediately following the death of a spouse are filled with continuous, stressful decisions and activities. From arranging a funeral and notifying family members and friends to dealing with finances and the sorrowing reactions of others, the surviving spouse has little time to rest or to think. The one advantage to the constant pressure is that the loss is not fully understood until after the funeral. It is during this period, reported a bereavement group of widows and widowers, that the surviving spouse will probably hear some thoughtless sentiments expressed by friends and family.

## Statements Heard by Surviving Spouses

*Helpful Remarks*

"Tell me how I can help."
"I'm so sorry."
"Tell me how you are."
"You are both always in
    my thoughts."

*Hurtful Remarks*

"Call me if there is
    anything I can do."
"He led a full life."
"I know how you feel."
"She's in heaven now."

The surviving spouse is instantly thrust into the task of building a new life. The shock caused by the loss of a wife or husband is powerful, and the work of building this new life is monumental. Without reasonably good health and dependable support systems, the possibilities of a satisfactory life in the future for the widow or widower are diminished.

The way people manage their grief and mourning may be influenced by their cultural traditions or by a role model such as a close relative or a prominent national personality. No matter how a bereaved person handles the process, he or she learns a number of new skills, however reluctantly. Life never is and never will be as it was before the death of the spouse, yet the widow or widower assumes this new identity with virtually no transition period.

The permanence of the loss of the relationship causes strong, visceral feelings experienced as pain and fear. A mourning process follows grief, and it is the external expression of these feelings in varying intensity. Some of the many factors contributing to mourning are the circumstances of the death, coping skills, spiritual beliefs, support of family and friends, and other life stresses.

A recently bereaved widow or widower is flooded with the emotions commonly associated with several phases of the mourning process. There is denial, frustration, and even anger at the powerlessness generated by the permanence of the situation. Mourners are chronically exhausted because of insomnia. Any feeling is legitimate, as the survival process is extremely hard work, always bewildering, always unavoidable.

Persons who have lost a spouse often question their own behavior. For example, Ellen's husband of forty years died after a prolonged illness, and she spoke of the comfort she received from wearing his old bathrobe at night. "It feels like his arms are around me, and it's very consoling, but I wonder if this is normal." When Burt's wife was admitted to a nursing home a few blocks from their home, it was a great convenience for him. Yet when she died, Burt would drive several blocks out of his way in order to avoid passing the facility. Different individuals use different coping skills. However, if daily tasks and routines are seriously inhibited by a behavior, it may be time to look for professional advice.

## Adapting to Life Without a Spouse

Prevailing social norms often inhibit the discussion of attitudes and feelings that surround dying and death. These taboos add to the shock of the loss and to the depression and despair that follow death. Furthermore, they can be major obstacles to the surviving spouse trying to get on with life.

A man who recently lost his wife joined a support group for the bereaved. He described his grief as "being in uncharted territory, without a map. I don't know where I'm going and I have no idea how to get there."

One of the most difficult steps toward living the "new" life of the surviving spouse is enduring the milestones that once were shared: the birthdays, anniversaries, and holidays. Situations such as these revive painful emotions. Members of bereavement support groups suggest having some plan well in advance of a special day, because it offers the survivor a measure of being in control rather than in the role of victim. Experienced widows and widowers recommend being with other people, such as family, friends, or members of other support groups. If the social interaction seems too stressful, a telephone visit may suffice.

Another problem mourners face is solo decision making. Married couples generally make major decisions after much discussion, weighing the advice and opinions of each other before reaching a conclusion. It is extremely risky to make major decisions alone during the first year after the death of a spouse. A move, a retirement, or a significantly different lifestyle usually should be postponed for a year after the death of a spouse. The passage of that one year allows time for increased perception and objectivity to develop in the recently widowed. There are always exceptions, however.

Don's wife died at home after a two-year illness. Just before Billie was diagnosed with cancer, they planned to sell the house and move into a retirement condo. All through the chemotherapy, Billie loved talking about the new life they would make together in the smaller, bright, modern condo. She persuaded Don to start packing most of their books and personal possessions long before they telephoned the movers. Even after the hospice team came in to care for her, she continually urged Don to carry on with the plans they had lovingly made together. Two weeks after Billie's death, Don moved.

"I'm not moving away from something," Don explained to his concerned son. "I'm moving toward something—my new life." Don's attitude and decision were right for him.

The negative feelings bereaved persons experience are very upsetting, despite reassurances that they are normal. Nevertheless, there are several ways of managing them: talking to a friend, writing in a journal, meditating, making a tape recording, and using spiritual resources often help during the mourning period. However, there still seems to be a general assumption that the widow or widower will "get over it"—that if the emotions of acute sadness and confusion (which the bereaved are encouraged and expected to display) are ventilated, they will ultimately be dispersed, and the mourner will "get on with life." Conversely, if the mourner does not show intensely sorrowful behavior such as crying, loss of appetite, or apathy, and then resumes a routine of activities, people assume the stage is being set for a poor emotional adjustment and inevitable psychological problems. However, grief is much more complex than that. First of all, there is no time limit on feelings of sadness, and second, the expression of feelings—whether in private or among friends—is only one part of the mourning process.

The reassessment of health practices after the death of a spouse promotes not only physical but emotional well-being. For example, balanced nutrition helps to control weight, maintain health, and increase energy. Extra energy provides for exercise, an important element in reducing tension and promoting sleep. (Some form of physical exercise is essential in order to reduce emotional stress.) Getting enough sleep boosts the immune system and improves overall health.

Widows and widowers generally agree that keeping busy with selected pleasurable activities, building a social life, and enhancing the homes in which they live, however simply, were all positive steps in the construction of their new lives. Moreover, taking control is rewarding. Maintaining autonomy increases self-esteem, builds confidence, and ensures a healthy psychological balance.

## Figure 9.2 Advance Directive for Patients

**My Durable Power of Attorney for Health Care, Living Will, and Other Wishes**

I, _____, write this document as a directive regarding my medical care.

Part I. My Durable Power of Attorney for Health Care

_____ I appoint the following person to make decisions about my medical care if there ever comes a time when I cannot make those decisions myself:

## Figure 9.2 Advance Directive for Patients (continued)

Name:_____ Tel: (H)_____(O)_____
Address: _____

_____

____ If the person above cannot or will not make decisions for me, I appoint the following person:

Name:_____ Tel: (H)_____(O)_____
Address: _____

_____

____ I have not appointed anyone to make health care decisions for me in this or any other document.

I want the person I have appointed, my doctors, my family, and others to be guided by the decisions I have made in Parts II and III below.

Part II. My Living Will

A.
1. ____ I do not want life-sustaining treatments (including CPR) started. If life-sustaining treatments are started, I want them stopped.
____ I want life-sustaining treatments that my doctors think are best for me.
____ Other wishes: _____

2. Artificial Nutrition and Hydration
____ I do not want artificial nutrition and hydration started if it would be the main treatment keeping me alive. If artificial nutrition and hydration are started, I want them stopped.
____ I want artificial nutrition and hydration, even if it is the main treatment keeping me alive.
____ Other wishes: _____

3. Comfort Care
____ I want to be kept as comfortable and free of pain as possible, even if such care prolongs my dying or shortens my life.
____ Other wishes: _____

B. These are my wishes if I am ever in a persistent vegetative state:

1. Life-Sustaining Treatments

\_\_\_\_ I do not want life-sustaining treatments (including CPR) started. If life-sustaining treatments are started, I want them stopped.

\_\_\_\_ I want life-sustaining treatments that my doctors think are best for me.

\_\_\_\_ Other wishes: _____

2. Artificial Nutrition and Hydration

\_\_\_\_ I do not want artificial nutrition and hydration started if it would be the main treatment keeping me alive. If artificial nutrition and hydration are started, I want them stopped.

\_\_\_\_ I want artificial nutrition and hydration, even if it is the main treatment keeping me alive.

\_\_\_\_ Other wishes:_____

3. Comfort Care

\_\_\_\_ I want to be kept as comfortable and free of pain as possible, even if such care prolongs my dying or shortens my life.

\_\_\_\_ Other wishes:_____

C. Other Directions

You have the right to be involved in all decisions about your medical care, even those not dealing with terminal conditions or persistent vegetative states. If you have wishes not covered in other parts of this document, please indicate them here.

_____

_____

_____

_____

_____

Part III. Other Wishes

A.

\_\_\_\_ I do not wish to donate any of my organs or tissues.

\_\_\_\_ I want to donate all of my organs and tissues.

\_\_\_\_ I want to donate only these organs and tissues:

_____

_____

Other wishes: _____

_____

_____

### *Figure 9.2 Advance Directive for Patients (continued)*

B. Autopsy

\_\_\_\_ I do not want an autopsy.

\_\_\_\_ I agree to an autopsy if my doctors wish it.

Other wishes: _____

_____

_____

Part IV. Signatures

Your Signature

By my signature below, I show that I understand the purpose and the effect of this document.

Signature: _____ Date: _____

Address: _____

Your Witnesses' Signatures:

I believe the person who has signed this advance directive to be of sound mind, that he/she signed or acknowledged this advance directive in my presence, and that he/she appears not to be acting under pressure, duress, fraud, or undue influence. I am not related to the person making this advance directive by blood, marriage, or adoption, nor, to the best of my knowledge, am I named in his/her will. I am not the person appointed in this advance directive. I am not a health care provider or an employee of the health care provider who is now, or has been in the past, responsible for the care of the person making this advance directive.

Witness #1

Signature: _____ Date: _____

Address: _____

Witness #2

Signature: _____ Date: _____

Address: _____

Source: Walter Reed Army Medical Center, 1996.

## *Figure 9.3 Personal Checklist for Documents and Instructions*

### Personal Checklist

Use the following personal checklist as a guide for identifying, collecting, and organizing important records, documents, and instructions. Use the Personal Inventory form on the next few pages to fill in more details about the documents and records that you have.

Personal checklist for: _____

(Name)

For a quick reference, place a check in the box next to the items that you have. You may have all, several, or just one or two of the items listed below. If you feel that some of the unchecked items may be important to you and/or your family, it may be helpful to talk with your family, doctor, clergy, lawyer, or insurance agent about the specific benefits of that item before making a decision.

- ☐ Birth certificate
- ☐ Social Security number
- ☐ Living will
- ☐ Durable power of attorney for health care
- ☐ Life insurance
- ☐ Health insurance
- ☐ Accident insurance
- ☐ Pension plan(s)
- ☐ Bank account(s)
- ☐ Safe-deposit box(es)
- ☐ Automobile(s)
- ☐ Real estate/rental papers
- ☐ Others

      _____

      _____

### Personal Inventory

Name _____

Date _____

Address _____

Date of Birth _____

### Figure 9.3 Personal Checklist for Documents and Instructions (continued)

Social Security Number _____

Next of Kin: Name _____

Next of Kin: Address _____

**Employer**
Name _____

Address _____

Company Benefits _____

**Personal Papers** (birth certificates, living will, etc.)
Location _____

Insurance Companies _____

     Life (Name and Policy Number)

     _____

     Automobile (Name and Policy Number)

     _____

     Other (Name and Policy Number)

     _____

Banking Papers (include pension plans, if any)

     Kind of Account, Bank Name/Address, Account Number.

     _____

     Kind of Account, Bank Name/Address, Account Number.

     _____

     Other Accounts (include Pension Plans and safe-deposit box(es)

     _____
     _____

Where _____

Account Number _____

Automobiles (make, model, year) _____

Real Estate Papers _____

**Personal Items of Value**

_____

_____

_____

**Counselors Who Can Help With My Affairs**
Attorney _____

Insurance agent _____
Doctor _____
Clergy _____
Other (broker, business associate, accountant)

_____

Funeral Arrangements

_____

_____

Special Requests

_____

_____

Source: National Cancer Institute, National Institutes of Health.

# 10

# Aging and Health Enhancement

ALONG WITH THE growth of the elderly population that began in the twentieth century, numerous health-related advances have resulted in the increased life expectancy of men and women. As a result, the present generation of older adults has survived longer than any other generation of elders before it. For the first time, the population includes extraordinary numbers of people in their seventies, eighties, and beyond who are physically fit and mentally active. This is the first group of older adults who have had access to superior medical technology and comprehensive health care. They are health- and fitness-conscious, and most of them have made changes in their lifestyles in order to enhance their health and well-being.

However, today's elderly population also has a number of concerns:

- The possibility of reductions in Medicare coverage
- The solvency of Social Security
- Costs of hospitalization and nursing home care
- Prescription drug expenditures
- The price of health insurance

These elders form a powerfully influential voting bloc—a force politicians do not underestimate. Increasingly, the large numbers of elderly will not only have expanded political and economic influence, but also, because of their diversity, will be a strong cultural influence that will enrich both older and younger adults.

Older adults' interest in their physical and mental health goes beyond acknowledging that a healthy lifestyle has beneficial effects. They want to learn how to achieve fitness and maintain optimum health.

Today's baby boomers—tomorrow's senior citizens—are a well-educated population and more socially active and politically involved than previous generations. They are receptive to change and will seek to develop, implement, and control the necessary changes. This group also expects to expect to live longer and more fully than adults of any previous generation.

## Health Behaviors and Lifestyle

Most older adults have a fairly good idea of the state of their own health. They understand the benefits of pursuing certain health-enhancing behaviors and activities, and they want to retain control over their lifestyle choices. In the mid-1980s, a group of older adults identified six health-promoting activities that they engaged in and perceived as important. In descending order of importance, they cited the following activities:

- Exercise
- Diet/nutrition
- Keeping busy
- Socializing
- Avoiding stress
- Visiting health professionals

We know that in the areas of nutrition, physical activity, alcohol consumption, and smoking, lifestyle governs the quality and length of life. Older adults understand that the choices they make in daily living are strongly linked to the state of their health. A healthy lifestyle is not a random occurrence. Rather, it results from two positive actions: protecting health and promoting health.

*Protecting health* means engaging in behaviors that decrease the chances of contracting illness or sustaining injury. For example, an older adult could protect his or her health by using preventive health services such as immunization clinics for the prevention of influenza or pneumonia, screenings for occult blood in the stool, prostate exams and mammograms, and blood pressure monitoring for hypertension. These services are for people who generally are healthy yet take seriously the responsibility for monitoring their own health.

*Promoting health* means focusing on diet, exercise, and other healthful activities. Most of today's elders are receptive learners, able to adapt the information required to meet their health care needs. They are eager and able to take the steps required to improve their physical fitness and nutritional awareness. Furthermore, older adults actively pursuing healthier lifestyles also make vigorous efforts to fulfill their potential for well-being. They learn to manage stress and to maximize their personal growth.

Doris, ninety-two, is a good example. She lived alone in a rural area, where she spent a lifetime successfully dealing with hardships, and she prized her endurance and independence. Her church activity and strong sense of spirituality gave her great comfort in rare moments of loneliness. When she fell and broke her hip, her family was pessimistic about her future. However, Doris survived not only the surgical repair but the serious complications that eventually left her unable to walk.

Reluctantly, her son admitted her to a nursing home. He, too, had health problems and was unable to care for her. After a few uncertain months adjusting to her newly imposed circumstances, Doris joined an activities program at the facility and took an immediate interest in both watercolors and ceramics. She said she enjoyed the color and the creativity. Her work was displayed in the nursing home's gift shop, modestly priced, and sold along with the other residents' crafts. When her first decorative bowl sold, Doris was delighted. It gave her a tremendous psychological lift.

Her son was very surprised at the development of this new hobby and her single-minded devotion to it. He never found her in her room; she was always in the activities workshop or monitoring sales in the gift shop. "Mother, I didn't know you even liked art. You never did anything like this before," he said, slowly shaking his head. "Well," said Doris, "maybe I never had the opportunity."

## Coping in Late Life

Just how do the elderly cope with the many obstacles and decrements normally encountered in old age? Many researchers in the field of geriatric psychology conclude that mental health and problem-solving skills are enhanced by remaining intellectually active as well as physically active. Successful older adults confront a problem by formulating some kind of plan. They are willing to accept new ideas and learn new techniques. These elders usually prevail in managing the more stressful life situations. Those who avoid or deny problems or resign themselves to a problem's outcome usually have a much less satisfactory resolution.

> *Many studies of elderly individuals indicate that successfully aging coincides with a lifetime of building successful relationships and achievements. Elderly research subjects shared a commonly held belief that remaining active allowed them to maintain some control over life events. They viewed challenges as a stimulus for growth.*

Effective age-related coping efforts are most common among people with higher socioeconomic status and education levels. Nevertheless, there is wide variation among individuals. Personal qualities associated with effective coping include stability, a good sense of self-esteem, and the power to make use of change so it works to one's advantage. Older adults say these qualities help them cope with late-life transitions.

# Creativity and Aging

Creative activity, that combination of emotion, imagination, and experience channeled into action, often flourishes in late life. Perhaps the urgency of being at the end of life stimulates creative expression. Another view is that older adults are less restricted by routine activities and obligations, so they have time and freedom to explore means of creative expression.

> *Keeping a journal stimulates mental activities. This practice allows for speculation, reinforces memory, develops observation, aids in problem solving, and encourages reflection.*

Many older adults who have pursued creative expression in art, music, or writing have noted that loneliness, a personal loss, or surviving a health crisis preceded their efforts in these areas. A typical example is keeping a journal. In recent years, writing in a journal has become a staple of self-help activity. Although it is unclear how or why "journaling" affects well-being, some psychologists believe that the immune system is improved by the reduction of negative emotions and intrusive thoughts. Furthermore, many revealed that the actual creative process was just as important as the emotional release journaling offers. Elders who engaged in this activity regained a sense of control because the daily routine of writing in a journal let them establish a sense of order within their disrupted lives. More important, they seized the opportunity to make something satisfying and positive after a loss or a period of depression.

Creativity is not limited to artistic expression. Any activity that is original and productive can be considered creative. Many opportunities for creative expression are available in the ordinary activities of daily life—for example, planning a meal, a meditation, or a day's activities. Being actively involved in a process is vital because this generates mental activity, and the physical effect on the body produces well-being and satisfaction. The ability to use imagination in order to develop an original process does not decline with age.

Elderly persons who view late-life transitions as opportunities stand the best chance of successfully managing the changes and losses that accompany aging. At times, they learn this viewpoint unwillingly, but mastering the inevitable physical and social setbacks offers huge returns in satisfaction and fulfillment.

As the number of older adults slowly but inevitably increases, it is essential to view these elders as a cultural resource. Their experience makes them valuable to younger people, their families, and their communities as role models, mentors, tutors, and contributors.

# Keeping the Mental Edge

At the age of sixty-eight, Margaret Mead, the noted anthropologist, was appointed a full professor and head of the social sciences department at Fordham University. Arturo Toscanini was eighty-seven when he made his last public appearance as a conductor. And when he was eighty-eight, Dr. Michael DeBakey, who pioneered the development of an artificial heart, went to Moscow to evaluate former Russian president Boris Yeltsin for open-heart surgery.

Were these just isolated instances of older adults living full and productive lives? Did they follow some special plan to ensure their cognitive competence? Why do we see that some individuals maintain their mental capacity, while others do not? Are there specific steps to take in order to avoid dreaded cognitive deficits?

Unimpaired brain function is a key requirement for enjoying old age. Older adults are appalled at the thought of developing Alzheimer's disease or some other form of dementia. Traditionally, Alzheimer's disease was considered a product of hereditary factors, while other dementias were thought to result from the depletion of reserves of active neurons in the aging brain. But recent investigations have demonstrated the ability of human brain tissue to generate new neuronal growth under laboratory conditions. This offers hope for promising treatments in the near future that will result in activating brain repair mechanisms.

We have some control over the likelihood of dementia. Studies indicate that the incidence of dementia decreases with the number of years of formal education. While these results are not conclusive, they do strongly suggest that older adults who engage in mental activity throughout their lives may unknowingly be protecting the neurons of their brains. In contrast, the passive practice of prolonged television watching by socially isolated elderly persons has been shown to add to their mental retrogression. Some researchers even regard it as a cause.

Other provocative research findings come from a singular investigation of dementia. A group of elderly nuns volunteered to participate in a research study of dementia. After their death, their brains were autopsied in order to clarify how the aging process influences the development of dementia. The reports showed that those who had a history of small strokes were ten times more likely to display symptoms of dementia than those who had no history of stroke. These results agreed with previous research findings that suggest a connection between stroke history and dementia. Such a link heightens the importance of nutrition's role in reducing the risk of stroke.

In some studies of memory and attentiveness, physical activity has been linked to cognitive function. The theory is that age-related cardiovascular changes and physical inactivity lead to hypoxia, or insufficient oxygenation of the brain. Aerobic exercise, which builds cardiovascular fitness, is said to improve the flow of oxygen to the brain and therefore impede the progress of cognitive declines.

# Managing Risks Associated with Aging

Although the longer life expectancy for babies born in the twenty-first century is unprecedented, several diseases remain linked to aging, chiefly arthritis, heart disease, and hypertension. In addition, the normal aging process is further associated with decline in bone density, decrease in muscle mass, reduction in strength, and increase in adipose tissue (body fat).

Adipose tissue increases from 18 percent of body mass in young men to 36 percent in elderly men, and from 36 percent in young women to 48 percent in elderly women. If the shift in body composition is unrestrained, some type of cardiac disease is virtually certain to develop. In fact, this often happens. The primary cause of death of all Americans is still traced to the cardiovascular system: heart disease and stroke.

However, a growing body of evidence confirms the influence of lifestyle and diet in successfully controlling fat increases and helping to ensure heart health. The correct balance of nutrition and regular physical activity will optimize the process of aging. Nutritional needs, the topic of Chapter 3, will be further addressed later in the chapter.

## Preventing Falls

One of the initiatives described in *Healthy People 2010* is the toll on older adults caused by fractures due to osteoporosis. Nearly 17 percent of women aged fifty and older and about 6 percent of men in that age group have osteoporosis, the loss of minerals in bone mass that leads to deteriorated and fragile bones.

Older adults can work on and improve bone density, muscle mass, and muscle strength. Ignoring these elements of good health produces the debilitating and often fatal consequences of falls.

Falls are a very serious geriatric public health problem. The elderly are hospitalized for fall-related injuries five times more often than they are hospitalized for injuries due to other causes. In addition, nearly one-third of elderly fall victims sustain injuries that dramatically reduce their mobility and independence and raise the risk of premature death.

There are also major economic consequences resulting from the aftermath of fall-related injuries. In 1996 the health care costs for fractures due to osteoporosis were estimated at $13.8 billion per year. That estimate did not take into consideration other significant consequences of injuries, such as disability and impaired quality of life. According to the National Center for Injury Prevention and Control, the total cost of all fall injuries for people aged sixty-five and older in 1994 was $20.2 billion. The center estimates that by the year 2020, the cost of fall injuries will reach $32.4 billion. Most often, these injuries are fractures of the hip, spine, or forearm.

Hip fractures are the most serious of the fall-related injuries in terms of subsequent health problems and fatalities. Half of all older adults hospitalized for hip fractures cannot return home or live independently after their injuries. The people most at risk are women and the oldest old. Women sustain 75 to 80 percent of all hip fractures. Persons eighty-five and older are ten to fifteen times more likely to experience hip fractures than are people between the ages of sixty and sixty-five.

Falls of elderly people were once viewed as unfortunate but unavoidable accidents. However, further investigation has revealed that in most cases it is possible to evaluate an older adult's potential for a fall and to take measures to reduce the chance of falls. Several factors influence the problem of falls by elderly persons who live in institutions and independently. Table 10.1 identifies causes related to the elderly person's physical condition and environment.

Older adults and their families need to take responsibility for reducing known hazards and maintaining a safe environment. Because 75 percent of falls occur in the home, the residence should be carefully evaluated for in-house dangers such as trailing electrical cords on the floor, cluttered traffic patterns, or stairways that need rails. Bathrooms are frequently the sites of falls. Handrails should be installed for bath, shower, and toilet use.

### Table 10.1 Common Causes of Falls

| Physical Causes | Environmental Causes |
|---|---|
| Neurological and musculoskeletal disabilities | Slippery surfaces |
| Medications that cause gait and balance disorders | Inadequate lighting |
| Dementia | Loose rugs |
| Visual impairments | Inappropriate footwear |
| Alcoholism | Objects or water on the floor |
| | Uneven flooring |
| | Unstable furniture |

Personal health maintenance is a critical step toward ensuring safety. Annual eye examinations and total medication evaluation by a health care provider can uncover elements that need correction or suggest interventions appropriate to reduce the risks of falls. Since falls are the sixth leading cause of death in persons over the age of sixty-five, and since they account for two-thirds of deaths in this age group, implementing safety strategies is critical. A program of regular exercise also can build the strength and stability that protect a person from falling.

# Exercise for Safety and Health

Elderly individuals should increase their physical activity by learning to structure an exercise program either alone or in a group. No one is too old to enjoy the benefits of regular exercise, which are improved strength, balance, and coordination. Of special interest to older adults is the evidence that muscle-strengthening exercise can reduce the risk of falls and fractures. This improves the ability to live independently and enhances lifestyle and well-being.

Strength training compensates for the age-related loss of muscle mass. It improves bone health, which reduces the risk for osteoporosis and improves posture and gait. Maximizing range of motion and flexibility also lowers the incidence of falls.

Regular participation in an exercise routine provides many psychological benefits, as well. Benefits identified through research include the lessening of depressive symptoms and concurrent behavior, improved feelings of self-worth and autonomy, and maintenance of cognitive function. In sum, the evidence is strong, both in physical and psychological terms, that regular exercise and activity foster independent living, expand functional capacity, and enhance the lifestyle of older adults.

Historically our society has taken the position that elderly people should be protected from doing physical tasks and encouraged to "rest." However, one of the healthiest things an older adult can do is to exercise and to increase physical activity—within reason—regardless of age. In fact, lack of exercise and adoption of a sedentary lifestyle usually cause physical and emotional damage. Participation in a regular exercise program prevents or reduces many of the functional declines related to old age.

Adopting healthier, more active lifestyles could permit most people to manage heart disease, the primary cause of hospitalization, disability, and death for those over sixty-five. Exercise can improve cardiac output by strengthening the heart muscle. A strong heart enhances the blood supply to all organs, thus improving their function. This maximizes independence and well-being in older adults.

*In the 1990s, researchers determined that barring genetic causes, lack of exercise and poor dietary habits are second only to smoking as the largest underlying causes of death.*

Many older adults mistakenly view exercise as an activity only for seniors who are in the younger age range, live independently, and can jog briskly or at least walk at a rapid pace. In fact, researchers have repeatedly demonstrated that exercise supplemented by strength training can improve the health even of people in their nineties. There is virtually no age limit. Just modest levels of regular physical activity are helpful. Even frail, elderly persons who have chronic diseases and who are disabled have benefited from exercise geared to their abilities.

*In the 1990s, studies of active centenarians found that most of them pursued healthy lifestyles by avoiding smoking, watching their weight, and exercising. The subjects also demonstrated a positive emotional outlook and the ability to manage the changes and losses their long lives inevitably brought. There was also an intriguing absence of any signs of Alzheimer's disease or other dementia.*

Formal exercise programs abound in senior centers and adult day-care settings, where the staff can monitor the progress of older adults. A popular program with older adults is tai chi, known to improve balance and flexibility. Tai chi is an ancient Chinese model composed of meditation and slow, repetitive movements. This and other exercise programs not only show participants how to increase endurance and strength but also how to maintain what they have achieved.

In very old people, even small gains can mean a big difference in developing and maintaining functional ability. Furthermore, the structured physical activity offered by formal exercise programs has benefits beyond physical health. These programs are excellent opportunities for expanding social contacts, developing independence, and increasing a sense of well-being.

All older adults should make daily exercise a routine. Research indicates that only about one-third of persons aged sixty-five and over reach recommended levels of physical activity. These recommendations range from vigorous physical activity aimed at achieving peak cardiorespiratory fitness to moderate levels of activity for improving general health.

> *Inactivity increases with age, especially among women. Inactivity is also more common among those with lower incomes and less education.*

Exercise differs from physical activity. A physical activity is any voluntary body movement that burns calories. Exercise is a physical activity that follows a planned format. It is a routine that consists of repeated movements with the goal of improving or maintaining one or more areas of physical fitness.

## Safety Issues

Before undertaking a new physical activity program, the elderly person should undergo a comprehensive physical evaluation by his or her primary health care provider. This is especially important for previously sedentary individuals, men over forty, women over fifty, anyone with a chronic disease such as a cardiovascular disorder or diabetes, and anyone at risk for those disorders.

After physician clearance for an exercise program, all participants need to observe commonsense safety precautions. For example, endurance routines should not cause breathlessness, dizziness, or chest pain. The routines should include the following elements:

- Warm up before doing a routine, and cool down afterward. A light activity such as walking at a comfortable pace is a good warm-up.
- Begin the exercise routine slowly, and increase the rate gradually.
- Stretch after the activity when the muscles are warm.
- Use appropriate safety equipment—for example, helmets when bicycling and suitable shoes when walking.

The aging body has diminished thirst sensation. To avoid dehydration, the older adult must replace fluids before experiencing thirst. This is especially important in hot weather or when perspiring.

Elderly individuals are more sensitive to temperature extremes. Too much heat can cause heatstroke, and exposure to very cold temperatures can lead to hypothermia.

Progress in any physical activity should be slow. When undertaking a new activity, the elderly person should gradually build up the time spent on the exercise routine, giving the body time to adjust. Later, the level of difficulty may be increased.

There are four types of physical activities: movements designed to build endurance, strength, balance, and flexibility. Each type of activity offers many health benefits for older adults.

## Endurance

Exercise for improving endurance—often called aerobic exercise—increases stamina by improving the health of the heart, lungs, and circulatory system. Activities that increase breathing and heart rate help to reduce the risk of developing heart disease and hypertension. Furthermore, research shows that aerobic activity improves the health of many older adults who already have those diseases. For example, endurance training for older adults with cardiovascular disease appears to be beneficial in the following ways:

- Blood pressure is lowered.
- Body weight and percentage of fat are reduced.
- LDL cholesterol (undesirable cholesterol) levels are lowered, and HDL cholesterol (desired cholesterol) is increased.

Body composition improves with endurance training similarly in younger and older adults. Also encouraging is the fact that aerobic routines of even low to moderate intensity appear to lower blood pressure in older hypertensive adults. Endurance exercises also can delay or prevent other age-related disorders such as diabetes, colon cancer, and stroke.

The prudent older adult who has been inactive for a long period of time should begin an exercise routine slowly. The goal is to gradually advance to a moderate to vigorous level that accelerates breathing and heart rate. The U.S. Surgeon General advises older adults to perform some type of thirty-minute activity that increases the breathing rate, three to five times a week. If thirty consecutive minutes are impractical, three ten-minute sessions can provide the same benefits. Table 10.2 lists examples of activities that can be part of an endurance exercise program.

### Table 10.2  Examples of Endurance Activities

| Moderate | Vigorous |
| --- | --- |
| Swimming | Swimming laps |
| Cycling | Shoveling snow |
| Walking briskly | Tennis (singles) |
| Golf without a cart | Skiing (cross-country and downhill) |
| Rowing | Climbing stairs or hills |

*Brisk walking is one of the safest and least expensive exercises for older adults. It requires no equipment (other than appropriate footwear) and places little stress on the knees and lower back. It is also one of the best activities for delaying or reversing the damage done by osteoporosis.*

## Strength Training

Muscle cells are made up of long strands of protein that lie close together. Muscle tissue can expand and contract. Strength training can build muscles, and even small increases in muscle bulk can boost the ability of frail elders to participate more independently in daily life activities.

Elderly persons lose from 20 to 40 percent of muscle mass as they age. However, researchers have found that the muscle is lost because of a reduction in physical activity, not just because a person has grown old. The sedentary lives of older Americans have become a cause of national concern. These findings emphasize the value and necessity of regular strength training. Regular practice of a strength-training routine can at least partially restore muscle mass and strength, even in very old people.

Most strength-training exercises are done with weights, starting with low levels of weights and repetitions and gradually increasing both. Progress is made by increasing the amount of weight used; the weight increases are usually made in small increments. However, some activities can be combined in order to build both endurance and strength. Examples of such combinations are walking uphill or raking leaves.

Even very small changes in muscle size can result in major gains in strength. But as strength increases, certain precautions must be observed in order to avoid injuries. For example, a minimum of weight should be used for the first week, and always warm up before a routine with light walking or arm pumping. After strength exercising, when muscles are warmed up, the person should also gently stretch the muscles. This stretching will help the person avoid injury.

## Stretching Tips

- Stretch *after* endurance and strength exercises, when muscles are warmed up.
- Hold the stretch position for ten to thirty seconds.
- Rotate the stretching routine to different positions and muscle groups.

To prevent injury during a strength-training routine, observe these safety recommendations:

- Maintain normal breathing patterns. *Exhale* during the stress portion of the exercise. Holding the breath and straining can cause dangerous changes in blood pressure.
- Following hip surgery, obtain clearance from the surgeon before embarking on a strength-training program.
- Use smooth, steady movements. Sudden, jerking movements can cause injury.
- Avoid locking leg or arm joints in a fixed position.
- When bending forward, bend from the hips, not the waist.
- Recognize the difference between muscle soreness and pain. Discontinue any exercise that causes pain. Muscle soreness, on the other hand, is normal and may last up to a few days.
- No exercise should cause exhaustion. In fact, most people who exercise regularly report an increase in energy and feelings of well-being.

A study of older adults with disabilities who participated in an in-home resistance training experiment yielded significant information. The subjects selected were put in an exercise program consisting of a five-minute warm-up, twenty-five minutes of strenuous exercise, and a five-minute cooldown. Participants could do the routine either standing up or sitting down. The researchers assessed the participants before they started the program, after three months of participation, and again after six months. The promising results of the research, described in the January 1999 issue of the *American Journal of Public Health*, indicated that home-based resistance exercise programs for older, disabled persons can provide measurable improvements in function.

## Balance and Flexibility Exercises

Each year 300,000 Americans are admitted to hospitals for broken hips, which are usually caused by falls. Balance and strength conditioning can help older adults avoid these falls and the threat of permanent disability and loss of independence. Conditioning exercises are designed to build up leg muscles in order to provide improved support and optimized equilibrium. Exercises done to strengthen the lower body also benefit the older adult by improving balance.

The balance exercises in Table 10.3 are all done while standing and holding onto a table or a chair with one hand. When comfortable with the balance exercise routine, the older adult can try holding on with one finger and then without holding onto anything for support.

### Table 10.3 Balance Exercises

| | |
|---|---|
| Plantar flexion | Stand on tiptoe. Slowly lower heels to the floor. |
| Knee flexion | Slowly bend the right knee so the right foot lifts up behind. Slowly lower the foot all the way down. Repeat with the left leg. |
| Hip flexion | Slowly raise the right knee toward the chest without bending the waist or hips. Slowly lower the leg. Repeat with the left leg. |
| Hip extension | Lean forward slightly at the hips, and slowly lift one leg (from the hip) behind you, keeping the leg straight. Slowly lower the leg. Repeat with the other leg. |
| Side leg raise | Slowly lift one leg to the side, raising it 6 to 12 inches above the ground. Slowly lower the leg. Repeat with the other leg. |

# Other Aspects of Health Enhancement

Optimizing health requires achieving a balance among several components of an older adult's lifestyle. Along with physical activity, just discussed, these components include exercise, nutrition, and the preservation of cognitive function.

## Meeting Nutritional Needs

The nutritional needs of older adults (as explained in Chapter 3) are vastly different from those of younger adults. The U.S. Department of Agriculture's Food Guide Pyramid does not fully show the nutritional needs of the aging adult. Therefore, the modified version of this guide, shown in Chapter 3, makes recommendations specific to the nutritional needs of the geriatric body.

Frank provides a good example of how nutritional needs change in the later years. He retired from his factory job when he was sixty-five, after working at the same plant for more than twenty years. Frank had eagerly looked forward to retiring. His friends at the plant professed to be envious about his getting to sleep late every morning and "take it easy" in general. Indeed, from a physical standpoint, Frank began to take it easy.

When he was employed, Frank used to walk a mile each morning and each evening to and from the public transportation that took him to work. Furthermore, his position as a supervisor required him to do a lot of walking. Upon retirement, Frank began to sleep late and to devote several hours a day to his only hobby, wood carving. Nights were spent watching TV or, more often, falling asleep in front of the set. In less than a year, Frank gained fifteen pounds.

Like Frank, most older adults have reduced energy needs because their activity levels are generally less than those of younger adults. Based on this change, the accepted daily standard for adults between fifty and seventy-five years of age need a 10 percent caloric reduction and an additional 10 to 15 percent after age seventy-five. To meet nutritional needs within these limits, the elderly person's diet should emphasize whole grains, fruits and vegetables, low-fat dairy products, and lean meat, fish, and poultry.

The Food Guide Pyramid for older adults also recommends eight cups of water daily. Water is essential for life, and most elderly do not get enough of it. Older adults are at risk for dehydration, because their thirst perception is dulled and their bodies have a far lower water content than those of younger adults. Also, the elderly consume many more medications, and some of these drugs interfere with the body's ability to regulate fluid balance. Not only does dehydration progress quickly in the elderly, but it also exacerbates the symptoms of constipation and kidney impairment.

One of the primary reasons elderly individuals limit their fluid intake is that they believe it is a way to reduce the number of trips to the bathroom, or chances of incontinence. However, in the long run, limiting fluids has just the opposite effect. Low fluid intake produces concentrated urine, which, in turn, irritates the bladder and may actually increase the need to urinate. Urinary tract infections often develop and may go unrecognized until the situation becomes serious.

## Older Adults and Smoking

Becoming physically fit requires more than dietary changes. Along with modifying diet and increasing exercise, elderly adults can improve their health by limiting alcohol and stopping smoking.

Older smokers are less likely than young smokers to try to quit. However, those who do try are more successful in their efforts than are younger smokers trying to quit.

Quitting smoking at any age offers substantial health benefits. However, the impact of smoking is more serious in older smokers, due to the cumulative effects of the habit. Thus, the risk of death and the chance of smoking-related diseases increases substantially as a person ages.

## Supplements

In their eagerness to embrace healthful living and achieve fitness, many older adults add supplements to their diets. Vigorous, persuasive marketing strategies imply that strength and vigor are available to anyone willing to buy so-called health food products. Although supplements are useful for persons who are unable to eat all the foods they need, a nutrient-dense balanced diet is still the best way for most older adults to meet their nutritional needs.

Although advertising messages aggressively tout the effectiveness of megadoses of many vitamin and mineral products, evidence of their benefits is usually only anecdotal. Furthermore, supplements are expensive. Many are even dangerous to ingest when consumed along with certain medications. Before taking any supplement, older adults should ask both their pharmacist and their health care provider the following questions:

- Does the supplement interact with the prescription drugs being taken?
- In what way is the supplement helpful?
- Is the supplement safe in the dose to be taken?

Always verify with a physician the wisdom of adding a supplement to a diet. Often, a diet based on the USDA's Food Guide Pyramid is enough to maintain optimum nutrition

## Satisfaction Strategies

Jacob, ninety-six, was a resident of an assisted-living facility. Asked what he thought were important factors in measuring his quality of life, the former librarian said, "Well, I'm glad that I can do most things for myself. I also enjoy talking to the folks around here, and I'm never lonely. There is always something going on or something to do. I play cards here a couple of times a week, and that's enjoyable."

Although Jacob outlived all of his family and most of his friends, he still regarded his life as meaningful. His outlook, despite some predictable physical declines, was positive. He looked forward to each day and, in fact, kept a running list of the activities he intended to participate in so he wouldn't forget to show up for them. Bridge was always on his list.

Generally, contentment with one's life in old age depends on having reasonably good health, financial security, and satisfying interpersonal relationships. However, many elderly also identify other areas such as spirituality, emotional growth, and a positive outlook on life as significant contributors to their well-being.

Life satisfaction is closely related to an individual's outlook. Mental decline that only a generation ago was believed to be inevitable was not at all evident in Jacob's interview. He challenged his mind with bridge, a game that demands concentration. (Word games and puzzles are other good mental activities.) Jacob also utilized lists and calendar reminders to help him remember what was important. He is social and engaging, and perhaps his lifelong personality traits helped in his overall adjustment to life as a very old man.

Negative, disruptive emotions such as anxiety, anger, or depression impede the ability to adapt to stressful environments and situations. Stress affects certain hormones that are involved in regulating the digestive system and the health of the skin. Stress also may damage a part of the brain that governs memory. Ways to reduce the stress response include a regular exercise program, including such alternatives as yoga. Biofeedback, another method of stress reduction, teaches control of stress responses.

The path to achieving a satisfying old age will vary for each individual. But most people who achieve this goal do so in three ways:

1. Maintaining fitness by participating in physical activity and eating a balanced, nutritious diet
2. Preserving cognitive function
3. Cultivating emotional stability in relationships

These strategies are available to almost any older adult. We all have the potential to succeed in managing the challenges of old age.

# Appendix A

# Eldercare Resources

AARP Fulfillment (funeral-related information)
601 East Street, N.W.
Washington, DC 20049
800-424-3410
www.aarp.org

AARP Widowed Persons Service
1909 K Street, N.W.
Washington, DC 20049
202-434-2260

Adaptive Devices
ABLEDATA (assistive devices)
8455 Colesville Road
Silver Spring, MD 20910
800-346-2742

Administration on Aging
U.S. Department of Health and Human Services
330 Independence Avenue, S.W.
Washington, DC 20201

Aging Network Services
4400 East West Highway
Bethesda, MD 20814
301-657-4321

Alcoholics Anonymous (AA)
475 Riverside Drive, 11th Floor
New York, NY 10115
212-870-3400

Alzheimer's Disease Education and Referral (ADEAR) Center
P.O. Box 8250
Silver Spring, MD 20907-8250
800-438-4380
www.alzheimers.org
24-hour toll-free hot line: 800-272-3900

American Association of Homes and Services for the Aging
7519 Connecticut Ave N.W.
Washington, DC 20008
202-783-2242
Fax: 202-783-2255

American Association of Retired Persons
601 E Street, N.W.
Washington, DC 20049
202-434-2120

American Dietetic Association
P.O. Box 97215
Chicago, IL 60678-7215
800-366-1655
www.eatright.org

American Psychiatric Association
1400 K Street, N.W.
Washington, DC 20005
888-357-7924
Fax: 202-682-6850
www.psych.org

Americans for Long-Term Care Security
1101 Vermont Avenue, N.W.
Washington, DC 20005
Fax: 202-682-3984
www.ltcweb.org

Asociacion Nacional Pro Personas Mayores
3325 Wilshire Boulevard, Suite 800
Los Angeles, CA 90010
212-487-1922

Assisted Living Facilities Association of America
9411 Lee Highway, Plaza Suite J
Fairfax, VA 22031
703-691-8100

Assisted Living Federation of America
10300 Eaton Place, Suite 400
Fairfax, VA 22030
703-691-8100
Fax: 703-691-8106

Better Hearing Institute
Hearing Helpline
P.O. Box 1840
Washington, DC 20012
800-327-9355

Center for Social Gerontology
2307 Shelby Avenue
Ann Arbor, MI 48103-3895
313-665-1126

Children of Aging Parents
1609 Woodburn Road, Suite 302A
Levittown, PA 19055
215-945-6900
800-227-7294

Choice in Dying
200 Varick Street
New York, NY 10014
212-366-5540

Concerned Relatives of Nursing Home Patients
P.O. Box 18820
Cleveland Heights, OH 44118
216-321-0403

Consumer Information Center (federal consumer publications)
Department WWW
Pueblo, CO 81009
888-878-3256
www.pueblo.gsa.gov

Consumer Response Center
Federal Trade Commission
600 Pennsylvania Avenue, N.W.
Washington, DC 20580
1-877-FTC-HELP (382-4357)
TDD: 202-326-2502
www.ftc.gov

Council of Better Business Bureaus, Inc.
4200 Wilson Boulevard, Suite 800
Arlington, VA 22203-1838
www.bbb.org
703-276-0100

Department of Veterans Affairs
Regional office information: 1-800-827-1000
www.ceu.va.gov

Eldercare Locator Hot Line
Administration on Aging (AOA)
1-800-677-1116 (9:00 A.M.–8:00 P.M. Eastern time, Monday
through Friday; voice mail after hours)
Note: Caller should be prepared with elderly person's address,
including zip code.

Foundation for Hospice and Home Care
320 A Street, N.E.
Washington, DC 20002
202-547-6586

Funeral Consumer Alliance
P.O. Box 10
Hinesburg, VT 05461
1-888-458-5563
www.funerals.org

Funeral Service Consumer Assistance Program
P.O. Box 486
Elm Grove, WI 53122-0486
800-662-7666

GriefNet (international computer link for those experiencing grief)
www.rivendell.org
E-mail: griefnet@falcon.ic.net

Health Care Financing Administration
7500 Security Boulevard
Baltimore, MD 21244
410-786-3000
www.hcfa.gov/about/agency

Hearing Aid Helpline
20361 Middlebelt Road
Livonia, MI 48152
800-521-5247

Hospice Association of America
519 C Street, N.E.
Washington, DC 20002
202-547-6586

Hospice Helpline
National Hospice Organization
1901 N. Moore Street
Arlington, VA 22209
800-658-8898

International Cemetery and Funeral Association
1895 Preston White Drive, Suite 220
Reston, VA 20191
800-645-7700
www.icfa.org

Jewish Funeral Directors of America
150 Lynnway, Suite 560
Lynn, MA 01902
781-477-9300
www.jfda.org

Judge David L. Bazelon Center for Mental Health Law (national
legal support for elderly people with mental disabilities)
1101 15th Street, N.W., Suite 1212
Washington, DC 20005-5002
202-467-5730

Knowledge Exchange Network (KEN)
800-789-2647
www.mentalhealth.org

Meals on Wheels Association of America
1414 Prince Street, Suite 202
Alexandria, VA 22314
703-548-5558
Fax: 703-548-8802
www.projectmeal.org
E-mail: mowaa@tbg.dgsys.com

Medicare Hotline
800-638-6833
800-492-6603 (in Maryland)

National Alliance for the Mentally Ill
Colonial Place Three
2107 Wilson Boulevard, Suite 300
Arlington, VA 22201-3042
703-524-7600; 800-950-NAMI
www.nami.org

National Association of Consumer Agency Administrators
www.nacaa.org/agencies.htm

National Association for Hispanic Elderly
3325 Wilshire Boulevard
Los Angeles, CA 90010
213-487-1922

National Association for Home Care
228 7th Street, S.E.
Washington, DC 20003
202-547-7424
Fax: 202-547-3540
www.nahc.org/home.htm

National Association of Professional Geriatric Care Managers
1604 N. Country Club Road
Tucson, AZ 85716
520-881-8008

National Bar Association (Black Elderly Legal Assistance Support
Project)
1225 11th Street, N.W.
Washington, DC 20001
202-842-3900

National Cancer Institute
Building 31, Room 10A24
Bethesda, MD 20892
800-422-6237

National Caucus and Center on the Black Aged, Inc.
1424 K Street, N.W., Suite 500
Washington, DC 20005
202-637-8400

National Center on Elder Abuse
1225 I Street, N.W., Suite 725
Washington, DC 20005
202-898-2586
Fax: 202-898-2583
E-mail: NCEA@nasua.org

National Center for Long Term Care
University of Minnesota School of Public Health
Institute of Health Services Research
420 Delaware S.E.
Box 197 Mayo
Minneapolis, MN 55455
612-624-5171

National Citizens' Coalition for Nursing Home Reform
1424 16th Street, Suite 202
Washington, DC 20036-2211
202-332-2275
Fax: 202-332-2949
E-mail: nccnhr@nccnhr.org (NCCNHR)
ombudcenter@nccnhr.org (Long-Term Care Ombudsman Center)

National Clearinghouse for Legal Services, Inc.
205 W. Monroe Street, 2nd Floor
Chicago, IL 60606-5013
312-263-3830

National Consumer Law Center, Inc.
11 Beacon Street
Boston, MA 02108
617-523-8010

National Council on Aging
409 Third Street, S.W.
Washington, DC 20024
202-479-1200
TDD: 202-479-6674
Fax: 800-424-9046

National Council on Alcoholism and Drug Dependence, Inc.
12 W. 21st Street, 8th Floor
800-NCA-CALL (800-622-2255)

National Council on Patient Information and Education
4915 St. Elmo Ave., Suite 505
Bethesda, MD 20814
301-658-8565
Fax: 301-656-4464
www.talkaboutrx.org
E-mail: ncpie@erols.com

National Depressive and Manic Depressive Association
730 N. Franklin, Suite 501
Chicago, IL 60601
www.ndmda.org
800-826-3632

National Elder Health Care Resource Center
University of Colorado at Denver
National Center for American & Alaskan Native Mental Health
Research
4455 East 12th Avenue, Room 308
Denver, CO 80220

National Family Caregivers Association
9621 E. Bexhill Drive
Kensington, MD 20895-3104
301-942-6430; 800-896-3650
Fax: 301-942-2302

National Federation of Interfaith Volunteer Caregivers
368 Broadway, Suite 103
Kingston, NY 12401
914-331-1358; 800-350-7438

National Foundation for Depressive Illness, Inc.
P.O. Box 2257
New York, NY 10016
212-268-4260; 800-239-1265
www.depression.org

National Funeral Directors Association
13625 Bishop's Drive
Brookfield, WI 53005
800-228-6332
www.nfda.org/resources

National Hispanic Council on Aging
2713 Ontario Road, N.W.
Washington, DC 20009
202-265-1288

National Hospice Organization
1901 N. Moore Street, Suite 901
Arlington, VA 22209
703-243-5900

National Indian Council on Aging
6400 Uptown Boulevard, N.E., Suite 510W
Albuquerque, NM 87110
505-888-3302

National Institute on Aging
Information Center
P.O. Box 8057
Gaithersburg, MD 20898-8057
800-222-2225
TTY: 800-222-4225
www.nih.gov/nia

National Institute on Alcohol Abuse and Alcoholism
6000 Executive Boulevard
Bethesda, MD 20892-7003
www.niaaa.nih.gov

National Institute of Diabetes and Digestive and Kidney Diseases
(NIDDK)
Office of Communications and Public Liaison
National Institutes of Health
31 Center Drive, MSC 2560
Bethesda, MD 20892-2560
www.niddk.nih.gov

National Institute of Mental Health
Information Resources and Inquiries Branch
6001 Executive Boulevard, Room 8184, MSC 9663
Bethesda, MD 20892-9663
301-443-4513
Fax: 301-443-4279
Depression brochures: 800-421-4211
TTY: 301-443-8431
FAX: 301-443-5158
www.nimh.nih.gov
E-mail: nimhinfo@nih.gov

National Insurance Consumer Helpline
800-942-4242

National Legal Assistance Support
American Bar Association
Commission on Legal Problems of the Elderly
1800 M Street, N.W.
Washington, DC 20036
202-331-2630

National Mental Health Association
1021 Prince Street
Alexandria, VA 22314-2971
703-684-7722; 800-969-6642
Fax: 703-684-5968
TTY: 800-433-5959
www.nmha.org

National Policy and Resource Center on Housing and
Long Term Care
University of Southern California
Andrus Gerontology Center
Los Angeles, CA 90089
213-740-1364

National Policy and Resource Center on Nutrition and Aging
Department of Dietetics and Nutrition, OE 200
Florida International University
University Park
Miami, FL 33199
305-348-1517
Fax: 305-348-1518
TTY: 800-955-8771
www.fiu.edu~nutrelder
E-mail: nutrelder@solix.fiu.edu

National Policy and Resource Center on Women and Aging
Brandeis University
Heller School–Institute for Health Policy
P.O. Box 9110
Waltham, MA 02254
617-736-3863

National Resource Center: Diversity and Long Term Care
Brandeis University
Heller School–Institute for Health Policy
P.O. Box 9110
Waltham, MA 02254
617-736-3930

National Resource Center on Native American Aging
University of North Dakota
P.O. Box 7090
Grand Forks, ND 58202-7090
800-896-7628

National Rural Long Term Care Resource Center
University of Kansas Medical Center
Center on Aging, 3901 Rainbow Boulevard
Kansas City, KS 66167-7117
913-588-1636

National Senior Citizen Law Center
1101 14th Street, N.W., Suite 400
Washington, DC 20005
202-289-6976
Fax: 202-289-7224
E-mail: nsclc@nsclc.org

National Stroke Association
96 Inverness Drive E, Suite 1
Englewood, CO 80112-5112
303-649-9299; 800-STROKES (800-787-6537)
Fax: 303-649-1328

Nutrition Hotline
American Dietetic Association
216 W. Jackson Boulevard, Suite 800
Chicago, IL 60606
800-366-1655

Older Women's League
666 11th Street, N.W., Suite 700
Washington, DC 20001
800-825-3695

Pension and Welfare Benefits Administration
U.S. Department of Labor
200 Constitution Avenue, N.W.
Washington, DC 20210
202-219-8871 (searching and locating documents)
202-219-8776 (questions about pension and health benefits)

Pension Rights Center
918 16th Street, N.W., Suite 704
Washington, DC 20006
202-296-3776

Social Security Administration
Office of Public Inquiries
6401 Security Boulevard, Room 4-C-5 Annex
Baltimore, MD 21235
800-772-1213
www.ssa.gov


Substance Abuse and Mental Health Services Administration
U.S. Department of Health and Human Services
www.samhsa.gov


USDA Center for Nutrition Policy and Promotion
1120 20th Street, N.W., Suite 200, North Lobby
Washington, DC 20036
202-418-2312
Fax: 202-208-2321
www.usda.gov/cnpp


U.S. Department of Agriculture
Food and Nutrition Information Center
14th Independence Avenue, S.W.
Washington, DC 20250
301-504-5719


U.S. Department of Health and Human Services
Administration on Aging
200 Independence Avenue, S.W.
Washington, DC 20201
202-690-6343 (HHS press office)
www.aoa.dhhs.govwww.hhs.gov/news/press (HHS press releases and
fact sheets)

U.S. Department of Health and Human Services
200 Independence Ave, S.W.
Washington, DC 20201
1-877-696-6775

Visiting Nurse Association of America
3801 E. Florida Avenue, Suite 900
Denver, CO 80210
800-426-2547

# Appendix B

# Government Clearinghouses

THE FOLLOWING LIST identifies specific clearinghouses maintained by the U.S. Department of Health and Human Services (HHS). For other sources of Health and Human Services information, see www.health finder.gov, accessible from the HHS website, www.hhs.gov.

Agency for Healthcare Research and Quality Publications Clearinghouse
800-358-9295; 301-621-3033
TDD: 888-586-6340

Alzheimer's Disease Education and Referral Center
800-438-4380

Low Income Home Energy Assistance Program Clearinghouse
888-294-8662

National Aging Information Center
202-619-7501
TTY: 202-401-7575

National Arthritis and Musculoskeletal and Skin Diseases
Information Clearinghouse
301-495-4484

National Clearinghouse for Alcohol and Drug Information
800-729-6686
TDD: 800-487-4890

National Clearinghouse for Primary Care Information
800-400-2742

National Diabetes Information Clearinghouse
301-654-3327

National Digestive Diseases Information Clearinghouse
301-654-3810

National Health Information Center
800-336-4797; 301-565-4167

National Institute on Deafness and Other Commmunication
Disorders Information Clearinghouse
800-241-1044
TDD/TTY: 800-241-1055

National Kidney and Urologic Diseases Information Clearinghouse
301-654-4415

National Mental Health Services Knowledge Exchange Network
800-789-2647

National Oral Health Information Clearinghouse
301-402-7364

National Women's Health Information Center
800-994-9662
TDD: 888-220-5446

Office of Alternative Medicine Clearinghouse
888-644-6226

Office of Minority Health Resource Center
800-444-6472; 301-587-9704 and 9705
TDD: 301-589-0951

Office of Population Affairs Clearinghouse
301-654-6190

Osteoporosis and Related Bone Diseases National Resource Center
800-624-2663

Weight-Control Information Network
800-946-8098

# Appendix C

# Websites for Caregivers

THE FOLLOWING DATABASES provide resources for housing, services, products for elder care (such as emergency response systems), and supportive chat rooms:

- www.caregiverzone.com
- www.careguide.com
- www.agenet.com
- www.aarplifeanswers.com

# Appendix D

# Suggested Readings

Albom, Mitch. 1998. *Tuesdays with Morrie: An Old Man, a Young Man, and Life's Lessons*. New York: Doubleday.

Billig, Nathan. 1987. *To Be Old and Sad: Understanding Depression in the Elderly*. Lexington, Mass.: D. C. Heath and Company, Lexington Books.

Bonder, Bette R., and Marilyn B. Wagner. 2000. *Functional Performance in Older Adults*. Philadelphia: F. A. Davis.

Brody, E. M. 1985. *Mental and Physical Health Practices of Older People*. New York: Springer.

Campbell, Scott, and Phyllis R. Silverman. 1996. *Widower: When Men Are Left Alone*. New York: Baywood Publishing Co.

Cumming, Elaine, and William E. Henry. 1961. *Growing Old*. New York: Basic Books.

Ebersole, Priscilla, and Patricia Hess. 2000. *Toward Healthy Aging: Human Needs and Nursing Response*, 5th ed. St. Louis: C. V. Mosby.

Eliopolous, Charlotte. 1997. *Gerontological Nursing*, 4th ed. Philadelphia: Lippincott Williams & Wilkins.

Ferro, K. F. *Gerontology: Perspectives on Aging*. New York: Springer Publishing Co.

Fitzgerald, Helen. 1994. *The Mourning Handbook*. New York: Simon & Schuster.

Hanks, Lela Knox. 1996. *Your Name Is Hughes Hannibal Shanks*. Lincoln, Neb.: University of Nebraska Press.

Hayflick, Leonard. 1994. *How and Why We Age*. New York: Ballantine Books.

Hooyman, Nancy R., and H. Asuman Kiyak. 1996. *Social Gerontology: A Multidisciplinary Perspective*. Boston: Allyn & Bacon.

Jackson, James S., ed. 1988. *The Black American Elderly: Research on Physical and Psychosocial Health*. New York: Springer Publishing Co.

James, John W., and Russell Freedman. 1998. *Grief Recovery Handbook*. New York: Harper Collins.

Kahn, Robert Louis, and John Wallis Rowe. 1999. *Successful Aging*. New York: Delacorte Press.

Kübler-Ross, Elisabeth. 1999. *On Death and Dying*. New York: Scribner Classics.

Lustbader, Wendy, and Nancy R. Hooyman. 1994. *Taking Care of Aging Family Members: A Practical Guide*, rev. ed. New York: Free Press.

Mace, Nancy L., and Peter V. Rabins. 1999. *The 36-Hour Day: A Family Guide to Caring for Persons with Alzheimer's Disease, Related Dementing Illnesses, and Memory Loss in Later Life*, rev. ed. Baltimore: Johns Hopkins University Press.

*Merck Manual of Geriatrics*, 3rd ed. 2000. Whitehouse Junction: Merck & Co.

Morris, Virginia. 1996. *How to Care for Aging Parents: A Complete Guide*. New York: Workman Publishing Co.

Nuland, Sherwin B. 1994. *How We Die: Reflection on Life's Final Chapter*. New York: Alfred A. Knopf.

Oliver, Rose, and Frances A. Bock. 1987. *Coping with Alzheimer's: A Caregiver's Emotional Survival Guide*. New York: Dodd, Mead & Co.

Perls, Thomas T., and Margery Hutter Silver with John F. Lauerman. 1999. *Living to 100: Lessons in Living to Your Maximum Potential at Any Age*. New York: Basic Books.

Roszak, Theodore. 1998. *America the Wise: The Longevity Revolution and the True Wealth of Nations*. Boston: Houghton Mifflin Co.

Sankar, Andrea. 1999. *Dying at Home: A Family Guide for Caregiving*. Baltimore: Johns Hopkins University Press.

Staudacher, Carol. 1987. *Beyond Grief*. Oakland: New Harbinger Publishing Co.

Teague, Michael L., and Richard D. MacNeil. 1992. *Aging and Leisure: Vitality in Later Life*, 2nd ed. Dubuque: W. C. Brown Communications.

# Appendix E

# Videos

THE AMERICAN ASSOCIATION of Retired Persons has produced a video-cassette titled *Survival Tips for New Caregivers*. The 1995 video includes a guidebook. To order, send $4 to AARP Program Resources Department, P.O. Box 51040, Washington, DC 20091.

Other videos dealing with aging and related issues are available from:

Terra Nova Films, Inc.
9848 S. Winchester Avenue
Chicago, IL 60643
800-779-8491; 773-881-8491
Fax: 773-881-3368
www.terranova.org

# Bibliography

Administration on Aging. *Profile of Older Americans*. U.S. Administration on Aging, 1999.

———. "The Elderly Nutrition Program." *Fact Sheet*, September 2, 1999.

Alzheimer's Association. "APOE Gene Testing." March 22, 2000.

Alzheimers.com. "Multi-Infarct Dementia (MID)." *Diagnosis*. PlanetRx, Inc., 2000.

American Association of Retired Persons (AARP). *Portrait of Older Minorities*. AARP Research Statistics Center, November 1995.

American Nurses Association. "Nutrition Screening for the Elderly," Position Statement. *Nursing World Reading Room*, December 11, 1992.

Andersen, M. L., and H. P. Taylor. "Age and Aging." *Wadsworth/ Thomson Learning* (Wadsworth Sociology Resource Center), February 29, 2000.

APA Online. "Disease Definition, Natural History, and Epidemiology." *Clinical Resources* (American Psychiatric Association).

Arnold, K. "Campaign for Patient Nutrition in Nursing Homes." *Family Practice News* 29(8), September 15, 1999, p. 7.

Ashok, and R. Ali. "The Aging Paradox: Free Radical Theory of Aging." *Experimental Gerontology* 34(3), June 1999, pp. 293–303.

Atchley, Robert C. "A Continuity Theory of Normal Aging." *The Gerontologist* 29(2), 1989, pp. 183–190.

Bachmann, Gloria A. "Sexual Dysfunction in Post Menopausal Women: The Role of Medical Management." *Geriatrics* 43, November 1988, p. 83.

Baker, F. M. "Mental Health Issues in Elderly African Americans." *Clinics of Geriatric Medicine* 11(1), pp. 1–3.

Becker, Gaylene. "Continuity After a Stroke: Implications of Life Course Disruption in Old Age." *The Gerontologist* 33(2), 1993, pp. 148–158.

Beers, M. H. "Explicit Criteria for Determining Inappropriate Medication Use in Nursing Home Residents." *Archives of Internal Medicine* 157, 1997, pp. 1,531–1,536.

Bell, Ronny A., and Kevin P. High. "Alterations of Immune Defense Mechanisms in the Elderly: The Role of Nutrition." *Top Nutrition Newsletter* 1(4), April 1998.

Bengston, V. L., and M. Silverstein. "Families, Aging and Social Change: Seven Agendas for 21st Century Researchers." In G. Maddox and M. P. Lawton, eds., *Annual Review of Gerontology and Geriatrics* 13, 1993, pp. 15–38.

Berger, Jeffrey T. "Culture and Ethnicity in Clinical Care." *Archives of Internal Medicine* 158, October 26, 1998, pp. 2,085–2,090.

Bernabei, R., G. Gambassi, K. Lapane, et al. "Management of Pain in Elderly Patients with Cancer." *Journal of the American Medical Association* 279(23), 1998, pp. 1,877–1,882.

Bernard, M. A. "Common Health Problems Among Minority Elders." *Journal of the American Dietetic Association* 97(7), 1997, pp. 771–776.

Blehar, Oren. "Gender Differences in Depression." *Medscape Women's Health* 2(3), 1997 (revised from "Women's Increased Vulnerability to Mood Disorders: Integrating Psychobiology and Epidemiology," *Depression* 3, 1995, pp. 3–12).

Blue, Amy V. "The Provision of Culturally Competent Medical Care." *Dean's Rural Primary Care Clerkship* (University of South Carolina), March 31, 2000.

Bootman, J. L., and J. A. Johnson. "Drug Related Morbidity and Mortality: A Cost of Illness Model." *Archives of Internal Medicine* 155(18), 1995, pp. 1,949–1,956.

Borgsdorf, Lawrence. "Improving Patient Compliance and Therapeutic Outcomes: Successful Models in Pharmaceutical Care." *On the Health Care Team* (Aventis), 2000.

Bortz, Walter M. "Sexuality and Aging: Usual and Successful." *Journal of Gerontology: Series A, Biological and Medical Sciences* 51(3), May 1996, pp. 142–146.

Brass, Lawrence. "Warfarin Underused in Elderly Stroke Patients." *Archives of Internal Medicine*, October 26, 1998.

Burstein, M. "Evolution and the Senescence Process: Broadening Our View of Aging." *Journal of Gerontologic Nursing* 24(9), September 1998, pp. 16–19.

Butler, Robert N. "The Viagra Revolution: Drug for Erectile Dysfunction Is Redefining Our Ideas About Sexuality Among Older Couples." *Geriatrics* 53(10), October 1998, p. 8.

Callahan, C., et al. "Health Services Use and Mortality Among Older Primary Care Patients with Alcoholism." *Journal of the American Geriatrics Society* 43(12), December 1995, pp. 1,378–1,383.

Carroll, Bernard J. "The Use of Antidepressants in Long Term Care and the Geriatric Patient: Geriatric Psychiatry Issues." *Geriatrics* 53, supplement 4, December 1998, pp. S4–S11.

Center for Disease Control and Injury Prevention. "The Costs of Fall Injuries Among Older Adults." January 27, 2000.

———. "Physical Activity and Health: A Report of the Surgeon General." November 17, 1999.

Chetkow-Yanoov, Benyamin. "Continuing Leadership Among Third-Age Professionals." Third European Congress in Gerontology, Netherlands Institute of Gerontology, 1995.

Chung, Ava. "Pilot Project to Identify Asian American and Pacific Islander Population's Health Care Needs." *Health Watch* (Department of Health and Human Services), June 1997.

Codispoti, Connie L., and Betty J. Bartlett. "Food and Nutrition for Life: Malnutrition and Older Adults." *Report by the Assistant Secretary for Aging*, Administration on Aging, Department of Health and Human Services, December 1994.

Cohen, A., et al. "Strategies to Protect Bone Mass in the Older Patient with Epilepsy." *Geriatrics* 52(8), August 1997, p. 70(6).

Cohen, Michael R. "Instituting Safe Medication Practices." *Conference of the American Pharmaceutical Association*, March 15, 2000.

*Consumer Reports on Health* 12(11), November 2000, p. 6.

Corti, M. C., et al. "Cardiovascular Diseases and Diabetes." *Women's Health and Aging Study*, National Institutes of Health, National Institute on Aging, 1995, p. 96.

Cronin-Stubbs, Diane, Carlos F. Mendes de Leon, et al. "Six-Year Effect of Depressive Symptoms on the Course of Physical Disability in Community Living Older Adults." *Archives of Internal Medicine* 160(20), November 13, 2000, pp. 3,074–3,080.

Davis, K., and S. Raetzman. "Meeting Future Health and Long Term Care Needs of an Aging Population." *Commonwealth Fund* Issue Brief, December 1999.

*Developments in Aging*, vol. 1. U.S. Senate Special Committee on Aging, U.S. Government Printing Office, Washington, D.C., 1997–1998.

Devine, Nancy. "American Natives Endure Increased Health Risks and Diminished Care." *NurseWeek/HealthWeek*, March 13, 2000.

*Diabetes in Hispanic Americans*, NIH Publication No. 99-3265. NIDDK, April 1999.

Dole, Ernest J., and Gireesh V. Gupchup. "A Review of the Problems Associated with the Screening Instruments Used for Alcohol Use Disorders in the Elderly." *Consultant Pharmacist* (American Society of Consultant Pharmacists), March 1999.

Evans, Gordon. "Sexuality in Old Age: Why It Must Not Be Ignored by Nurses." *Nursing Times* 95(21), May 26, 1999, pp. 46–47.

Ferriolli, E., et al. "Aging, Esophageal Motility, and Gastroesophageal Reflux." *Journal of the American Geriatrics Society* 46, 1998, pp. 1,534–1,537.

Fischer, Joan, and Mary Ann Johnson. "Low Body Weight and Weight Loss in the Aged." *Journal of the American Dietetic Association* 90, 1990, pp. 1,697–1,706.

Fouts, M., and J. Hanlon, "Medication Related Problems in Older Adults." *American Society of Consulting Pharmacists* 12, 1997, pp. 1,103–1,111.

Gabany, J. M. "Factors Contributing to End of Life Care." *Journal of the American Academy of Nurse Practitioners* 15(11), November 2000.

Gage, Barbara, and Thy Dao. "Medicare's Hospice Benefit: Use and Expenditures." Cohort U.S. Department of Health and Human Services, Office of Disability, Aging and Long Term Care, 1996.

Gants, R. "Detection and Correction of Underweight Problems in Nursing Home Residents." *Journal of Gerontological Nursing* 23(12), December 1997, pp. 26–31.

Gates, J., and Walter Rogers. "Minimization of Medication Misadventures." *Successful Models in Pharmaceutical Care: On the Health Care Team* (Aventis Pharmaceuticals), 2000.

George, Asha M. "Improving Influenza and Pneumococcal Immunization Among High Risk Adults." Summary, National Coalition for Adult Immunization, October 1998.

Glass, T. A., et al. "Change in Productive Activity in Late Adulthood: MacArthur Studies of Successful Aging." *Journal of Gerontology* 50(2), 1995, pp. 565–576.

Goldstein, S., et al. "Biologic Theories of Aging." *American Family Physician* 40(3), September 1989, 195–200.

Gordon, S. M., and S. Thompson, "The Changing Epidemiology of Human Immunodeficiency Virus Infection in Older Persons." *Journal of the American Geriatric Society* 273(20), May 1996.

Gottlieb, Stephen B., Robert J. McCarter, and Robert A. Vogel. "Effect of Beta-Blockade on Mortality Among High-Risk and Low-Risk Patients After Myocardial Infarction." *New England Journal of Medicine* 339(8), August 20, 1998, pp. 489–497.

Grady, Patricia A. *Statement on Improving Care at the End of Life: Research Issues.* House Committee on Government Reform, October 19, 1999.

Graedon, Joe, and Teresa Graedon. "Viagra Deaths Underscore Drug Interaction Dangers." *The People's Pharmacy/Health Central*, June 8, 1998.

Grant, W. B. "Dietary Links to Alzheimer's Disease." *Alzheimer's Disease Review* 2, 1997, pp. 42–45.

Gruman, Gerald J., ed. "Roots of Modern Gerontology and Geriatrics." *F. D. Zeman's Medical History of Old Age*. New York: Arno Press, 1979.

Grymnpore, R. E., P. A. Mitenko, D. S. Sitar, et al. "Drug Associated Hospital Admission in Older Medical Patients." *Journal of the American Geriatric Society* 36, 1988, pp. 1,092–1,098.

Guigoz, Yves, et al. "Nutrition Surveys in the Elderly: Assessing the Nutritional Status of the Elderly." *Nutrition Reviews* 54(1), January 1996, 559–565.

Gupta, Krishan. "Sexual Dysfunction in Elderly Women." *Clinics in Geriatric Medicine* 6(1), February 1990, pp. 197–199.

Gurwitz, J. H., and J. Avorn. "The Ambiguous Relation Between Aging and Adverse Drug Reactions." *Annals of Internal Medicine* 114(11), 1991, pp. 956–966.

Habel, Maureen. "The Oldest Old: A New Gerontological Challenge." *NurseWeek/HealthWeek*, July 13, 1998.

Hill, Steve M., and Alma M. Saddam. *Food Guide for African Americans*, Senior Series 172-00. Ohio State University Extension, Department of Aging, 1999.

Horgas, A. L., and P. F. Tsai. "Analgesic Drug Prescription and Use in Cognitively Impaired Nursing Home Residents." *Nursing Forum* 47(4), July/August 1998, pp. 234–241.

Hugo, Graeme. "Asian Population Studies," Series No. 141. University of Adelaide, Australia, April 2000.

Jette, Alan M., Margie Lachman, Marie M. Giorgetti, et al. "Exercise—It's Never Too Late: The Strong-for-Life Program." *American Journal of Public Health* 89(1), January 1999, pp. 66–72.

Jones, B. A. "Decreasing Polypharmacy in Clients Most at Risk." *AACN Clinical Issues* 8(4), 1997, pp. 627–634.

Katz, P. O. "Gastroesophageal Reflux Disease." *Journal of the American Geriatrics Society* 46, 1998, pp. 1,558–1,565.

Katzman, R., and C. Kawas. "The Epidemiology of Dementia and Alzheimer's Disease." In *Alzheimer Disease*, edited by R. D. Jerry, R. Katzman, and K. L. Bich. New York: Raven Press, 1994, pp. 105–122.

Keay, Timothy J., and Ronald S. Schonwetter. "Hospice Care in the Nursing Home." *American Family Physician*, February 1, 1998.

Kemp, Charles. "Hispanic Cultures: Mexican and Mexican-Americans." Clinical Notes, Baylor University, 2000.

Kligman, E. W. "Office Evaluation of Sexual Function and Complaints." *Clinics in Geriatric Medicine* 7(1), February 1991, pp. 15–39.

Krumholz, Harlan M. "Elderly Heart Attack Patients Often Denied Clot-Dissolving Drug Treatment." *Journal of the American Medical Association* 277, 1997, pp. 1,683–1,688.

Kuhn, D., and A. Ortigara. "The Growing Challenge of Alzheimer's Disease in Residential Settings." Rush Alzheimer's Disease Center, National Institute on Aging, and Alzheimer's Disease Education and Referral Center (ADEAR), 1999 (slides).

Kurtzweil, Paula. "Staking a Claim to Good Health." *FDA Consumer* (U.S. Food and Drug Administration), November–December 1998.

Laferriere, Rita H., and Brenda P. Hamel-Bissell. "Successful Aging of Oldest Old Women in the Northeast Kingdom of Vermont." *Image* 26(4), Winter 1994.

Laflin, Molly T. "Promoting the Sexual Health of Geriatric Patients." *Topics in Geriatric Rehabilitation* 11(4), 1996, pp. 43–54.

Lopez, C., and F. Aguilera. "On the Sidelines: Hispanic Elderly and the Continuum of Care," Publication q8. National Council of La Raza, February 1991.

Lynne, Joanne, et al. "Perceptions by Family Members of the Dying Experience of Older and Seriously Ill Patients." *Annals of Internal Medicine* 126, January 15, 1997, pp. 97–106.

Mackel, Cindy, et al. "The Challenge of Detection and Management of Alcohol Abuse Among Elders." *Clinical Nurse Specialist* 8(3), 1994, pp. 128–134.

Malugani, Megan. "Failing the Elderly." *NurseWeek*, January 27, 2000.

"Maximizing the Effectiveness of Drug Therapy in the Elderly." *Educational Software* (Columbia Presbyterian Medical Center), 1997.

Mayo Clinic Health Oasis. "New Procedures for GERD." *Ask the Mayo Physician*, June 12, 2000.

Mazzeo, Robert S., Peter Cavanaugh, William Evans, et al. "Exercise and Physical Activity for Older Adults." *Medicine and Science in Sports and Exercise* 30(6), June 1998, pp. 992–998.

McCorkle, Ruth, et al. "Effects of Home Nursing Care for Patients During Terminal Illness on the Bereaved's Psychological Distress." *Nursing Research* 47(1), January/February 1998, pp. 2–9.

McKenna, Matthew T., Eugene McCray, and Ida Onorato. "Epidemiology of Tuberculosis Among Foreign Born Persons in the United States." *New England Journal of Medicine* 332(16), April 20, 1995, pp. 1,071–1,076.

McLaughlin, Thomas J., and Jerry H. Gurwitz. "Delayed Thrombolytic Treatment of Older Patients with Acute Myocardial Infarction." *Journal of the American Geriatric Society* 47(10), October 1999.

McLeod, Peter J., Allen R. Huang, Robyn M. Tamblyn, et al. "Defining Inappropriate Practices in Prescribing for Elderly People: A National Consensus Panel." *Canadian Medical Association Journal* 156(3), 1997, pp. 385–391.

Mellinger, B. C., and J. Weiss. *American Urology Association Update Series*, no. 11, 1992.

Miller, Douglas K., et al. "Total Quality Management and Geriatric Care." Keynote Address, World Congress of Gerontology, International Association of Gerontology, 1997.

Mojon, P., et al. "Relationship Between Oral Health and Nutrition in Very Old People." *Age and Aging* 28(5), September 1999, pp. 463–468.

Morrison, R. Sean, and Albert L. Siu. "Survival in End Stage Dementia Following Acute Illness." *Journal of the American Medical Association* 284(1), July 5, 2000, p. 47.

Mui, A. C. "Self-Reported Depressive Symptoms Among Black and Hispanic Frail Elders: A Sociocultural Perspective." *Journal of Applied Gerontology* 12(2), 1993, pp. 170–181.

National Aging Information Center. *Malnutrition and Older Americans*. National Aging Information Center, Florida International University, March 2000.

National Council of LaRaza. *Hispanic Elderly*. Washington, D.C.: National Council of LaRaza, March 2000.

National Institute of Mental Health. "Older Adults: Depression and Suicide Facts," NIH Publication No. 99-4593.

———. "If You're over 65 and Feeling Depressed: Treatment Brings New Hope," NIH Publication No. 96-4033.

National Institutes of Health. "A Consumer's Guide to Mental Health Services," NIH Publication No. 94-3585.

———. "Depression," NIH Publication No. 99-3561, November 1999.

———. "Exercise: A Guide from the National Institute of Aging," NIH Publication No. 99-4258.

National Institute on Aging. "Exercise: Feeling Fit for Life." *Age Page*, 1998.

———. "Aging and Alcohol Abuse." *Age Page*, 1995.

———. "Forgetfulness: It's Not Always What You Think." *Age* p.1006.

———. "Alzheimer's Disease Fact Sheet." *Alzheimer's Disease Publications*, ADEAR Center, August 1995.

———. *Progress Report on Alzheimer's Disease 1999*, NIH Publication No. 00-4664. National Institute on Aging, National Institutes of Health, ADEAR Center.

National Stroke Association. "Stroke Prevention Guidelines." National Stroke Association, 1999.

National Women's Health Information Center (NWHIC). "Factors Affecting the Health of Women of Color." *Women of Color Health Data Book*. NWHIC, February 10, 2000.

Neel, Armon B. "Comorbid Disorders: Anxiety and Depression in the Nursing Home Resident." *Journal of the American Society of Consultant Pharmacists* 11(4), 1996.

"New Program Raises Diabetes Awareness Among Native Americans." *Diabetes Forecast* 53(1), January 2000, p. 66.

Norrgard, Carolyn, Carol Matheis-Kraft, and Sally Rigler. "Dementia." *Clinical Reference Systems*, July 1, 1999, p. 409.

Nowrojee, S., and J. Silliman. "Asian Women's Health: Organizing a Movement." *Dragon Ladies: Asian American Feminists Breathe Fire.* South End Press, 1997.

"Nutrition and Dementia." *Food and Nutrition Resource Newsletter* (Human and Environmental Sciences Extension's Resource) No. 96-5, September/October 1996.

O'Hare, William P. "A New Look at Poverty in America." *Population Bulletin* 51(2), September 1996.

"Older Americans 2000: Key Indicators of Well-Being." Federal Interagency Forum on Aging-Related Statistics, July 28, 2000.

Onega, L. L., and T. Tripp-Reimer. "Expanding the Scope of Continuity Theory." *Journal of Gerontological Nursing* 9(2), 1997, pp. 16–19.

Pareo-Tubbeh, Shirley L., et al. "A Comparison of Energy and Nutrient Sources of Elderly Hispanic and Non-Hispanic Whites in New Mexico." *Journal of the American Dietetic Association* 99(5), May 1999, pp. 572–582.

Passel, Jeffrey S., and Barry Edmonston. "Immigration and Race in the United States: The 20th and 21st Centuries," Government Documents Reference JV6463. Washington, D.C.: The Urban Institute, 1992, p. 36.

Ponza, Michael. *Serving Elders at Risk: Older Americans Act Nutrition Programs, National Evaluation of the Elderly Nutrition Program, 1993–1995.* U.S. Department of Health and Human Services, 1996.

Proctor, Jennifer. "Palliative and End-of-Life Care: A Course Requirement for Doctors-in-Training?" *Reporter* 9(3), December 1999.

Rabins, P. V., et al. "Outreach Program Effective in Identifying and Treating Elderly Experiencing Psychiatric Symptoms." *Journal of the American Medical Association* 283, June 7, 2000, pp. 2,802–2,809.

Rajogopalan, Shobita, and Deborah Moran. "Tuberculosis in Older Minority Adults." *Clinical Geriatrics Magazine Online* 6(7), July 1998.

Reuters Medical News. "Malnutrition, Dehydration in U.S. Nursing Homes Pinned on Staffing Problems." Reuters, June 9, 2000.

Richardson, J. P. "Sexuality and the Nursing Home Patient." *American Family Physician* 51(1), January 1995, pp. 121–124.

Rigler, Sally K., Stephanie Studenski, and Pamela W. Duncan. "Pharmacologic Treatment of Geriatric Depression: Key Issues in Interpreting the Evidence." *Journal of the American Geriatric Society* 46, 1998, pp. 1–5.

Rohleder, Wendy M. "Alcohol and Drug Abuse Among the Elderly." *Kansas Elder Law Network*, December 15, 1999.

Roubenoff, Ronenn. "The Pathophysiology of Wasting." *Journal of Nutrition* 129 (American Society of Nutritional Sciences), 1999, pp. 256s–259s.

Rowe, John W. "Successful Aging." Keynote Address, 75th Anniversary Symposium, Harvard School of Public Health, 1997.

Russell, Robert M., et al. "Modified Food Guide Pyramid for People over Seventy Years of Age." *Journal of Nutrition* 129 (American Society for Nutritional Sciences), 1999, pp. 751–753.

Ruth, Jan-Erik, and Peter Coleman. "Personality and Aging: Coping and Management of the Self in Later Life." In J. E. Birren and K. Warner Schaie, eds., *Handbook of the Psychology of Aging*, 4th ed. San Diego Academic Press, 1996, pp. 308–321.

Salvatore, T. "Elder Suicide: A Gatekeeper Strategy for Home Care." *Home Healthcare Nurse* 18(3), March 2000, pp. 180–186.

Satcher, David. "Mental Health: A Report of the Surgeon General." 2000.

Sciavi, R. C., and J. Rehman. "Sexuality and Aging." *Urology Clinics of North America*, 1995.

"Serving Elders at Risk." *Older Americans Act Nutrition Program*. Princeton, N.J.: Mathematica Policy Research, Inc., 1996.

Shearer, Gail. "Prescription Drugs for Medicare Beneficiaries: 10 Important Facts." *Consumers Union*, April 14, 2000.

Shell, Judith A., and Colleen K. Smith. "Sexuality and the Older Person with Cancer." *Oncology Nursing Forum* 21, 1994, pp. 553–558.

Shelton, Deborah L. "6 Myths About the Elderly." *American Medical News* 39(9), March 4, 1996, p. 6.

Silver, Marjorie Hutter, and Thomas T. Perls. "Is Dementia the Price of a Long Life? An Optimistic Report from Centenarians." *Journal of Geriatric Psychiatry*, Spring 2000.

Smith, Sidney C. "Ace Inhibitor Therapy: Benefits and Underuse." *American Family Physician* 59(1), January 1, 1999.

Soumerai, Stephen B. "Adverse Outcomes of Underuse of Beta Blockers in Elderly Survivors of Acute Myocardial Infarction." *Journal of the American Medical Association* 277(2), January 8, 1997, pp. 115–121.

Spagnoli, A., et al. "Drug Compliance and Unreported Drugs in the Elderly." *Journal of the American Geriatric Society* 37(7), 1989, pp. 619–624.

Standridge, John. *Alcohol Abuse in the Elderly*. Department of Family Medicine, University of Tennessee, November 1998.

Steinweg, Kenneth K. "The Changing Approach to Falls in the Elderly." *American Family Physician* 6(7), November 1, 1997.

Strehler, Bernard Louis. "Genetic Instability as the Primary Cause of Aging." *Experimental Gerontology* 21, 1986, pp. 283–319.

Stuck, A. E., and M. H. Beers. "Inappropriate Medication Use in Community Residing Older Persons." *Archives of Internal Medicine* 154, October 10, 1994.

Sullivan, D., et al. "Protein Energy Undernutrition Among Elderly Hospitalized Patients: A Prospective Study." *Journal of the American Medical Association* 281(21), June 2, 1999.

*Taber's Cyclopedic Medical Dictionary*, 18th ed. Philadelphia: F. A. Davis Publishing Co., 1997.

Tennstedt, S. "Family Caregiving in an Aging Society." *Longevity in the New American Century*, Baltimore, Md.: U.S. Administration on Aging Symposium, March 29, 1999.

Teri, Linda, et al. "Behavioral Treatment of Depression in Dementia Patients: A Controlled Clinical Trial." *Journal of Gerontology: Psychological Sciences* 52B(4), 1997, pp. 154–166.

Tichy, Anna M., and Marie L. Talashek. "Sexually Transmitted Diseases and Acquired Immunodeficiency Syndrome." *Nursing Clinics of North America* 27, 1992, pp. 937–949.

Tofani, Loretta. "A Nursing Home Alternative: Foster Care." *Philadelphia Inquirer*, May 23, 2000.

Torres-Gill, F. M. *Malnutrition and Older Americans*. Department of Health and Human Services, Administration on Aging, National Aging Information Center, April 5, 2000.

U.S. Bureau of the Census. "Sixty-Five Plus in the U.S." *Statistical Brief*, May 1995.

———. "Poverty Statistics on Population Groups." *Current Population Survey*, March 1996.

U.S. Bureau of the Census and National Institutes of Health. "Profiles of America's Elderly: Racial and Ethnic Diversity of America's Elderly Populations," POP/93-1. Washington, D.C., U.S. Government Printing Office, 1993.

U.S. Department of Agriculture. "The Nutrition Safety Net: Help for the Elderly and Disabled." *Primer for Enhancing the Nutrition Safety Net for the Elderly and Disabled*, July 14, 1999.

U.S. Department of Health and Human Services. "Depression in the Elderly," Fact Sheet. Public Health Service, Alcohol, Drug Abuse and Mental Health Administration.

———. *On Mental Health Issues*. Fact Sheet, December 13, 1999.

U.S. Department of Health and Human Services, Office on Women's Health. "Factors Affecting the Health of Women of Color: Elderly Women of Color." *Women of Color Health Data Book*. National Women's Health Information Center, 1995.

Vieira, Suzanne. "Multicultural Counseling Tips: Food for Thought and Action." *ADA's Courier*, November/December 1998.

Webster, R. Tim. "Total Drug Therapy Cost Control: A Comprehensive Vision of Consultant Pharmacy's Expanding Role in Health Care." American Society of Consulting Pharmacists, May 1996.

Weddle, D. O., et al. "Incorporating Nutrition Screening in Three Older Americans Act Elderly Nutrition Programs." *Journal of Nutrition for the Elderly* 17(1), 1997, pp. 19–37.

Weiss, Jeffrey N., and Brett C. Mellinger. "Sexual Dysfunction in Elderly Men." *Clinics in Geriatric Medicine* 6(1), February 1990, p. 188.

Whitfield, Keith E. "Study of African-Americans Finds Clues to Successful Aging." *Ethnicity and Disease*, November 1997.

Whooley, M. A., et al. "Depression, Falls, and Risk of Fracture in Older Women." *Archives of Internal Medicine* 159, March 8, 1999, pp. 484–490.

Williams, J. W., et al. "Primary Care Physicians' Approach to Depressive Disorder." *Archives of Family Medicine* 8, 1999, pp. 58–67.

Wisensale, S. K. "World Population Aging: The Coming Intergenerational Debate." *Bulletin on Aging*, No. 2/3 (U.N. Division for Social Policy and Development), 1997.

Womack, Pam, and Carolyn Breeding. "Position of the American Dietetic Association: Liberalized Diets for Older Adults in Long Term Care." *Journal of the American Dietetic Association*, 1998, pp. 201–209.

Yeates, Conwell, et al. "Completed Suicide Among Older Patients in Primary Care Practice: A Controlled Study." *Journal of the American Geriatrics Society* 48, 2000, pp. 23–29.

Zarit, S., and E. E. Femia. "Predicting Changes in Activities of Daily Living: A Longitudinal Study of the Oldest Old." *Journal of Gerontology: Psychological Sciences*, November 1997.

# Index